"At a time when outcome validity and cost dominat of us who work with spec personal stress and introspection and, at times, [illegible] focus of special education in general. The complexity and enormity of the educational challenge to serve children with severe disabilities can cause educators, therapists and administrators to lose sight of the value and dignity of each life entrusted to their care. Robert Greenwald's book, *My Son, My Gentle Son,* is a heart rending story of a precious life that, although very short, permanently impacted all who shared that life, and continues to awaken a sensitivity, compassion and sense of purpose in anyone who has a special child in their life. As the reader journeys through David's short life with his father, Robert Greenwald, he or she focuses anew on what really matters in the work that we do and evokes sympathy and understanding for the families of special children. Educators, therapists and school administrators who allow the raw emotion and simple truths of David's life and his family's experiences to penetrate their own lives will be more effective in the work they do. David's life, then, continues to grow in the depth of its influence and meaning."

Gretchen Kennedy, P.T.
Physical Therapist
Akron Public Schools

"With his words, Robert Greenwald paints a portrait of the profound and perfect love that develops when a family chooses to cherish the gift of their child's life. In rich detail he describes the daily rituals of family life with such honesty, such intensity, it almost took my breath away.

Above all else, this is the story of love—a love so rare, so pure, that it triumphs even after the life itself is gone.

Every word wrapped itself around my parent heart—and tugged."

Mimi Hunt
Mother of a child with disabilities

"Mr. Greenwald's book is a must-read for professionals who work with families of children with special needs. It is thought-provoking and brings the important feelings of parents into focus! Every early intervention professional should read this and infuse what they've read into everyday practice in their work with families."

Bethany Shue, M.S.A., M.A.
Past Clinical Audiologist
Current Training and Education Manager
Ohio Department of Health
(Ohio's lead agency for early intervention)

"I have used Robert Greenwald's book in my special education teacher preparation class at the University of Akron for the past three years. While our university students are required to read many texts, there is none more powerful and touching than *My Son, My Gentle Son.* Reading this book facilitates the type of empathy, understanding and caring that is essential for effective teaching. My students have consistently reported that reading and discussing the book has been one of the most powerful and influential activities they have encountered during their undergraduate or graduate training. They have also stated that they wish all educators were required to read this book as part of their teacher preparation programs.

I am grateful for the development of such a wonderful and influential book. Through it, little David continues to touch the hearts of others and contribute to their growth as future educators and individuals.'

Evonn Welton, Ph.D.
Assistant Professor
Department of Special Education and Counseling
University of Akron

"*My Son, My Gentle Son* has become required reading for the graduate course in family-professional collaboration. The powerful story of David and his family captures the attention of students in ways that no traditional textbook alone can do. Students have shared that they have laughed, they have cried, and they have walked away with a significantly deeper understanding of the journey faced by families when they have a child with a disability. Such an understanding cannot help but prepare students to be more effective, thoughtful educators and collaborators with families."

Marilyn Espe-Sherwindt, Ph.D.
Family Child Learning Center
Kent State University

My Son, My Gentle Son

My Son, My Gentle Son

Robert Greenwald

People with Disabilities Press,
Stanley D. Klein, Ph.D., Series Editor
iUniverse, Inc.
San Jose New York Lincoln Shanghai

My Son, My Gentle Son

All Rights Reserved © 2001 by Robert Greenwald

People with Disabilities Press,
Stanley D. Klein, Ph.D., Series Editor
iUniverse, Inc.
an imprint of iUniverse.com, Inc.

For information address:
iUniverse.com, Inc.
5220 S 16th, Ste. 200
Lincoln, NE 68512
www.iuniverse.com

ISBN: 0-595-17426-4

Printed in the United States of America

For David,
my gentle son

February 16, 1979 - August 16, 1987

"My somber heart seeks you always..."

Pablo Neruda

Several poems in this book have been previously published in *Kaleidoscope: International Magazine of Literature, Fine Arts and Disability* as follows: "Artist Unknown", volume 12, Winter, 1986; "The Silent Ringmaster", volume 14, Winter/Spring, 1987 and again in volume 19, Summer/Fall 1989; "Where I Stand", volume 19, Summer/Fall, 1989.

"The Silent Ringmaster" was also published in *Exceptional Parent Magazine*, November/December, 1993.

My love and gratitude to Barb, my partner, my companion on this journey. Thanks for your support, your encouragement, your memories. There are easier roads to travel, but none so fulfilling.

Thanks to the following people:

Stanley Klein, Editor, People With Disabilities Press; Jerry Mahoney, for believing in this project and bringing it to its original publication; Kay Greenwald, for computer and technical assistance in the preparation of the manuscript; Mimi Hunt, James May, Jane Nichols and Mary Beth Rollick for thoughtful criticisms and ideas, as well as their encouragement; Kathy Wilson, for her expertise in formatting the manuscript; LouAnne Greenwald for her cover illustration. Again, a special thanks to James May for his generous offer to write the foreword to this book.

FOREWORD

The old myths are far flung -- and deeply held -- that men are hard-driven, inexpressive, pragmatic creatures, devoid of strong emotions or the capacity to nurture, always more at home with work than with their families. Whatever truths such stereotypes might contain are shattered by Robert Greenwald's reflections of his son. For all parents a child's birth is a time of great expectation, joy and optimism. In David Greenwald, born with congenital heart disease that lead to subsequent brain damage, such dreams are crushed. Perhaps the easy choice would have been to turn away, abandon hope, and fatalistically accept life's injustices. For Robert that simply would not do. With eloquence he unabashedly shares with us the connections he creates with his son: the tears and depression, the fears and the pain, and ultimately, the love and care grounded in the extraordinary relationship they develop.

Reading *Gentle Son* evoked potent feelings in me. I often found myself twisting and turning at the raw emotions, so very close to the bone. In a narrative that is heart-rending, without being maudlin or sentimental, it explores the profound changes wrought by tragedy and grief. Having dealt with thousands of fathers of children with special needs, I can say with certainty that Robert Greenwald has spoken deep, fundamental truths. For parents and families who have suffered the loss of a child in death or in life, and for professionals who deal with such families, *Gentle Son* lends understanding to the painful, conflicting emotions associated with loss and with parenting a special child. It also lends hope and encouragement. There is an authenticity here that cannot be denied. This is a story not only to be read, but *felt*.

James May
Program Director
National Fathers' Network

TABLE OF CONTENTS

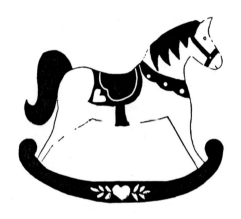

Chapter
One

"I'm afraid this child will not make you very happy."
a pediatric neurologist, after disclosing our son's diagnosis

"Bob. Wake up, Bob!"

I was sound asleep when I heard my wife, Barbara, summoning me awake, her hand shaking my shoulder.

"What? What's the matter?"

"Look, I'm wet. My water broke."

"Are you sure? Maybe you just wet yourself."

"No way! This is it—we're going to have a baby today! Come on, we'd better shower and get dressed and go to the hospital!"

"Are you in pain?"

"No. We don't have to rush."

It was 6:00 in the morning, February 16, 1979. As I rolled out of bed and put my feet on the floor, her words echoed in my mind— "This is it." This was the day we'd been waiting for and preparing for. This was the day we would become a family. The more I awakened, the more incredible it seemed: in a matter of hours, I would become a father—forever.

Barb and I had been married about two years when we decided—or, more accurately, when she decided—it was time to start a family. I was employed as a produce manager for a supermarket chain and Barb was a clerical worker for a division of General Motors. I was somewhat hesitant, for reasons both real and vague, about having a child. We were living in a rented twinplex at the time. I felt it would be more practical to buy a home before we began thinking about parenthood. And the added responsibilities of fatherhood—whatever they were—made me a little nervous. Not that I was opposed to the idea of familyhood; in fact, I had come from a family of ten, Barb from a family of five. During our courtship and early marriage we often daydreamed and talked together about how idyllic our lives would be: *our* love, *our* children, *our* home. Life could do us no wrong. Looking back, I recognize the bonding that took place between us in those shared, important dreams. We were young, naive lovers excited to be at the threshold of the most thrilling, most commonplace adventure of life: marriage and family.

I had eventually come around to accepting the idea of having a baby, and even became proud of Barb's pregnancy, perhaps in the egotistical way of most expectant fathers. In the meantime, we had found the house we wanted and we bought it. We spent the following months painting, wallpapering, remodeling, and making ready a room for our baby.

Today, that dreamed-of baby would become a reality—in our eyes, in our arms, and in our hearts. We showered and dressed. I ate a little breakfast while Barb packed a suitcase, and by 9:30 we were at the hospital. Barb was admitted. I was detained to fill out the customary forms and paperwork.

Barb and I had been going through the training and practice sessions for natural childbirth in the past few months. We looked forward to sharing this experience together. In a short time now, I would be trying out my abilities as her "coach." But first, I was directed to a locker room, where I was given the traditional green sterile surgical uniform to put on before entering the labor room. While changing clothes, I took from my pocket a printed "handout" sheet and drilled myself on the breathing exercises that Barb would be using.

As I entered the labor room I saw Barb lying on the bed, looking pale. She had been "prepped", that is shaved, enemized and IV'd -- aspects of the childbirth experience she had not fantasized about. Now she was feeling tired, but her labor had begun full force after the doctor inserted a long needle to fully puncture the amniotic sac. I stood beside her and held her hand. She made a remark about how silly I looked in my green costume. The next nine hours were long and painful ones as Barb's labor intensified. I tried to comfort her and engage her in conversation as much as possible, but she was constantly distracted by the pains.

We had chosen the name David if the baby was a boy, and Sarah, if a girl. At one point during the labor, I looked down at Barb and asked "David? or Sarah?" "Just healthy", she grunted. At this point, the pain was becoming unbearable for her. When the baby finally began to crown, she was instructed to hold it back while they administered a saddle-block anaesthetic and wheeled her into the delivery room. There, the actual birth began. I was so excited I was shaking! I could feel the adrenalin pumping through me. Barb began pushing on cue, while I held her hand, wiped her forehead, and mimicked the breathing exercises with her. Soon, the baby's head emerged; then, a shoulder, a fist, an arm, and in seconds, it was completely out.

"It's a boy!" the doctor informed us. I walked closer to make a visual assessment of him as they were cleaning him off. Everything was there — including his cry. I turned and gave Barb the "OK" sign, and she beamed. I smiled back at her. For a few moments we were both suspended in a kind of quiet glow—the sheer mystery and sense of wonder that follows the witnessing of such a miracle. Everything that biology and science courses had taught us about the human body, everything we had studied and learned in preparation for this event somehow fell short now of explaining what we had just seen. The two of us had created this new life. Our son. Our offspring. It was an event that both humbled us and exalted us; a reality that left us in awe and astonishment. We will never forget it.

After cleaning him and swaddling him snugly in a blanket, a nurse placed him in Barb's arms, where we said the first hello to our David, welcoming him into the world.

"He looks a little blue," Barb commented.
"They all do," said the nurse, overhearing her, "but they pinken up in a while."
"Can I unwrap his blanket?" Barb asked.
"You certainly may. He's your baby," she responded with a whimsical smile.

We took turns holding him, studying him from head to toe and commenting on his features. We narrated the dreams we had for him and the possibilities life would hold for him, sometimes exaggerating them to the point of laughter. It was all so wonderful—too wonderful to believe that having a baby was such a universal, commonplace experience.

At work the next day I was proudly announcing the birth of my son and passing out "It's a Boy" cigars and mints to fellow employees. All were congratulating me. Then, I received a phone call. It was from Barb.

"Hi!" I answered cheerfully, "How are you feeling" How's our little pup?"

"Bob," she said, "there's a problem. Can you come to the hospital?"

Her voice was cracking. I could tell she was on the verge of tears.

"Honey, can you talk? What's the matter?"

"They...they're taking the baby to the children's hospital," she sobbed, "because his color is still a little bluish, and it gets worse when he cries or sucks. And when our pediatrician came to examine him this morning, she detected a heart murmur."

"What does all that mean? What is the doctor saying?" I asked, hearing my own voice trembling now.

"I'm not sure. She'll explain it to us when you get here. Please hurry."

"I will," I assured her.

At the hospital, the nurse brought David to Barb's room so we could see him before he was transported to the children's hospital. I hadn't seen him since the day before. He looked so tiny and helpless. Barb held him in her arms and spoke to him softly while her eyes filled with tears. This isn't the way things were supposed to go, I was thinking. David is supposed to be a perfect, healthy baby. That's how we planned it. Now, they're carting him away to another hospital for tests on his heart. Who knows what they'll find? Our doctor said that many children are born with unexplainable heart murmurs that disappear as they grow older. But her concern stemmed from the combination of both a heart murmur and the "cyanotic" coloring of David's skin.

So he was transported to the local children's hospital for testing. There, a pediatric cardiologist, after evaluating David, concluded that surgery might be necessary. A hole that appears in every infant's heart at birth, but gradually begins to close shut thereafter, was doing just that — closing up prematurely and causing David's body to get less oxygenated blood. That hole would have to be opened wider, requiring either a heart catheterization or surgery. Since the hospital did not have a pediatric heart surgeon on staff, David was transported to another children's hospital about 40 miles away.

Barb wanted so badly to be with David, to follow him, to be there for him through every step of every procedure. But she would be confined to the hospital for the next four days. The geographical distance between her and David was relatively slight, but the tug of motherly instinct made that distance seem immense. I drove up to the other hospital with my parents the following day to speak to the cardiologist after a heart catheterization was performed.

"We were able to expand the opening by using a catheter with a tiny balloon-like apparatus on the end of it," he said." Therefore, we did not have to perform surgery immediately. However, the reason your child requires that hole to remain open is that he has a serious congenital heart disease."

He sat me down at a table and drew a simple diagram of the heart, showing the left and right sides, each with its upper and lower chambers.

"Your son's condition is called tricuspid atresia," he explained. "That's a term we use to describe an underdevelopment of the valve between the upper and lower chambers. It exists on the right side of your son's heart—the side that pumps blood to the lungs to

7

pick up fresh oxygen. But the valve problem is further enhanced by the fact that this lower right chamber is severely underdeveloped. Therefore, his body is not getting a normal amount of oxygenated blood. And that is why he has a dusky, bluish pallor, especially in his lips, fingers and toes."

Much of his explanation made sense to me as I recalled studying about the heart and lungs in high school biology. In fact, my biology instructor was born with a three-chambered heart, and had the same bluish-grey pallor to his features.

"What about his brain?" I asked. "Is it getting enough oxygen?"
"Yes, it is. And as far as his physical activity goes, you won't have to restrict him. He will limit himself: that is, when he becomes fatigued or short of breath, he will automatically stop or slow down whatever he is doing."

The cardiologist wanted to keep David there in the hospital for further tests and observation. He said that surgery had not yet been ruled out as a possibility.

After driving back home with my parents, I returned to the hospital where Barb was staying to share all of this information with her. We were shocked and saddened to know that our baby had a serious congenital heart disease. Barb even began to feel guilty. She searched through the past nine months wondering what she might have done to cause this condition in our baby. Was it that bee sting, she wondered. Had she over-exerted herself fixing up the new house? Had she not eaten properly? She desperately wanted some reason, some explanation for why our child was not perfect. I tried to reassure her that it was not caused by anything she did or did not do. We would probably never know the cause. The worst thing she could do, I told her, was to blame herself. There might be more crises ahead of us, and to allow some unfounded guilt to overwhelm her would only make all our lives more difficult. The prospect of possible surgery made us extremely nervous. But at this point, all we could do is wait it out, hoping and praying that surgery would not be necessary.

Two days later Barb was released from the hospital. She could not wait to see David. Before we left home to drive the forty miles up to the hospital, she packed an overnight bag, planning to stay at his bedside. When we arrived at the hospital we had a conference with the cardiologist. He informed us that he intended to release David that day. Barb and I looked at each other with a sense of great relief.

Then he continued, "However, he will definitely require some kind of corrective or constructive surgery further down the road, two to six months, perhaps, depending on his growth. But for now, he's not a good candidate for such surgery because he's so tiny. It would be far too risky."

He hooked us up with a cardiologist at our local children's hospital who, along with David's pediatrician, would monitor his condition closely and on a regular basis. That afternoon was the unexpected, but joyful, homecoming: Barb and I and our new son, all together. Over the next few days, in-laws, relatives and friends came to see him and bring gifts. Our house was full of pride and happiness.

In the weeks that followed, we began adjusting to our new roles and to the changes in schedule and in lifestyle they brought with them. We enjoyed holding David, feeding him, bathing him, and talking to him. Already he was growing and changing. At three weeks, he began taking a little diluted cereal from a spoon. This was prescribed by the pediatrician in hope of putting some weight on him for the possibility of surgery. By now, he was looking at us when we spoke to him. A few weeks later, we experienced the thrill of his first smile. And, of course, there were the customary snapshots: David in each new outfit, David in my arms, David in Barb's arms, David with his grandparents, David in any pose or activity we could imagine. It was all so new that we couldn't seem to stop taking pictures!

On Thursday, March 30, Barb and David and I went to a family gathering at my parents' house. Both my older brother and my older sister, who lived out of town, were home for a few days. It was a happy occasion having all ten members of our family gathered together in one place. We took pictures of some of the family members holding David, and some of David side-by-side with his cousin Kevin, born two months earlier to my older brother and his wife. These were the first two grandchildren in the family, so they drew a lot of attention. Everyone, too, was interested in hearing about David's condition. I can remember comparing the two infants in my own mind that evening and feeling somewhat cheated, somewhat jealous, perhaps, that my nephew was so whole and healthy, free of the kind of problems that David had. Why couldn't our son be blessed with the same good fortune, I wondered.

That evening David exhibited some strange behavior. He seemed alternately lethargic, then extremely fussy. I couldn't be sure if his color was bluer than usual, or if it was just my imagination. Then Barb pointed something out to me that we had not seen him do before: he rolled his eyes upward and held them there for several seconds, as if in a trance, then returned them to their normal position. We didn't know what to make of it, but decided he was tired. So we said our goodbyes and went home and tucked David in for the night. He slept soundly.

At work the following morning, I received a phone call. It was Barb.

"Bob, I'm at the pediatrician's office with David. An ambulance is on the way to take us to the children's hospital."

"What happened?" I asked, in shock.

"David slept straight through the night and on into the morning. He's never slept that long! I began to get worried so I woke him up at ten o'clock. He began crying uncontrollably and nothing I did would calm him down. His color looked bad and his breathing seemed erratic. I...I couldn't be sure, so I brought him here. The doctor says he's in respiratory failure! She has an oxygen mask on him right now. Oh..here's the ambulance. Meet us at the hospital, okay?"

When I arrived at the hospital emergency room, a nurse informed me that my son had been admitted to the intensive care unit. I rode the elevator up to the floor she directed me to. As I entered the room, I saw Barb standing in the foreground with her back to me. She was staring at the bustle of activity in front of her. A doctor and several nurses were gathered around an isolette containing our son. They had fastened the electrodes of a monitor to his chest. I stood beside Barb and held her hand, while we watched David's little belly ballooning in and out as he labored for breath. Several times he stopped breathing altogether, until a nurse reached into the isolette and thumped him on the chest with the flick of a finger. It was a pitiful and terrifying drama we were watching, unable to do anything to help him. Watching the movements of the doctor and nurses, hearing the grave tone of their voices as they spoke to one another in medical jargon, and seeing our son struggling inside of that plexiglass box sparked a fear in me that was nothing short of panic. "My God," I thought, "is he dying?" Finally, a doctor asked us to wait out in the lounge while they tried to stabilize him. Some time later he came out to talk to us.

"You have a very sick baby," he said. "His heart has malfunctioned, causing him to go into respiratory failure. His blood oxygen level is low. We're giving him pure oxygen now to keep him going. But, he needs to have emergency heart surgery. Since we don't have a pediatric heart surgeon on staff, he'll have to be transported to another children's hospital. Our cardiologist has spoken to their cardiologist, and arrangements have been made for surgery. Our biggest concern is getting him there quickly enough. We'd like to send him by helicopter, but they don't have a landing facility there. So our only choice is to send him by ambulance, with a nurse and a respiratory technician on board to manually "bag" him with oxygen. He'll be leaving shortly. But I have to be honest with you: I wouldn't be surprised if he literally died on the way—he's just that sick."

There was that word —"sick". Suddenly it had taken on a new meaning to me. In my own mind, "sick" had always been a word to describe some transitory illness—cold, flu, chicken pox, etc. Now it was used to describe the failed heart inside my son's body that was threatening his life, a reality far beyond my own experience and comprehension of sickness. I don't know what word I would have used, but "sick" seemed desperately inappropriate.

Barb's father drove us up to the hospital. It was the same one David had been transferred to only weeks before. My older brother and sister rode along with us. A close friend, who was also David's godmother, drove up later to join us.

After a long wait, Barb and I were finally permitted to see David. They had not yet performed surgery on him. When we entered the intensive care unit, we were jarred by the sight of our baby framed in a maze of tubes, wires and hardware. His little arms and legs were fastened to the bed sheets with restraints. Glued to his chest were the electrodes of a heart monitor. In his mouth was the hose from a respirator which, at regular intervals, inflated his chest. Inserted into his head was an IV needle. In his wrist were two more tubes: one was an IV; the other, a direct tap into his artery for drawing or injecting blood. His eyes were closed. Seeing him "wired" and fastened to all of this equipment heightened not only the reality of his condition, but our overwhelming fear of what could ultimately go wrong. We were suspended in a state of shock, dread and anguish. We were as helpless as our son. Everything was out of our hands now. We stayed at his bedside touching him and talking to him for about a half hour, then returned to the waiting lounge.

A short while later, the surgeon came to talk with us. He was a tall, lanky man dressed in green surgical garments, and he had a pair of adjustable scopes fastened to his eyeglasses. He began by asking us a few questions about David. Then he explained what had happened to David in the last 24 hours, how serious it was, and the surgical procedure he would be using to "correct" it. It sounded like an intricate technical procedure demanding a high level of surgical skill and knowledge. He warned us that the most dangerous part of the operation would be the anesthetic: there were no guarantees that David's heart could handle a general anesthetic. But if it could, he reassured us, David's chances for survival were about 90%.

The next few hours were spent waiting for the outcome. The six of us sat in the lounge and alternated between conversation and a kind of fearful, prayerful silence. Time passed slowly, each minute surrendering to the next in a tedious, protracted span that seemed like eternity. And through it all I don't think any of us stopped thinking of David for even a moment. In our own hearts and minds we, too, were waging the fight for his life. I kept thinking of the surgeon's projection for David's chances of survival — 90%. How strange, I thought, how ironic that we measure the ratio between life and death by percentages, the same standard we use for predicting the chances of rainfall or return on investment. Did he pull that figure — 90% — out of the air, or was it exact? I could not know. But I wanted to believe there was some infallible congruity between mathematical principles and his skilled hands.

"Why is this taking so long?" Barb asked. "It's been two hours."

That was the same question I had been asking myself, fearful that something had gone wrong. Barb and I were both tired. Our stomachs were in knots. Our nerves were frayed. We were shoring up everything inside of us in the name of hope, and the work was exhausting. With no one nearby to answer them, the questions became more persistent.

Finally, at about midnight, the surgeon entered the waiting lounge. He sat down at a table with us.

"David's surgery," he told us, "seems to be successful. Initially, we were uncertain of the outcome. It seemed that the procedure had not taken hold and we might have to open him up again. But as it turned out, that was not necessary. His heart is now circulating well-oxygenated blood. The next twenty-four to forty-eight hours will be the true test. If the surgical procedure continues to hold, and if his blood gas levels continue to improve, then David is free and clear of danger."

"Can we see him now?" Barb asked.
"Certainly," he replied.
As he walked us down the corridor, he added, "You'll notice a difference in his color."

When we entered the intensive care unit we saw David, his tiny chest wrapped in surgical bandages, still breathing with the respirator and still surrounded by tubes and wires. But there was one important difference: he was, for the first time, pink in color. That dusky, blue color he had since birth, especially in his lips, toes and fingertips, was gone. It was replaced by that healthy pink blush most babies are blessed with. Though he was still asleep, we stayed by his bed for a long while just staring at him. We were looking at a miracle. Relief and joy were welling up inside us, bringing tears to our eyes.

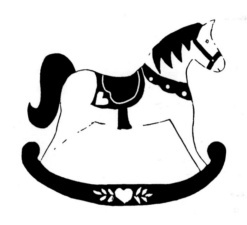

Chapter
Two

After his surgery, David was moved to the cardiac recovery unit of an adjacent hospital. The only infant in the unit, he was strapped to an adult-sized bed. He looked so small and out-of-place. A man in another bed across the room who was also recovering from heart surgery was old enough to be David's great grandfather!

Several times a day they took blood samples from David and analyzed them for levels of oxygen and other components. His condition was being closely monitored and was showing improvement. Barb was spending the nights at the hospital so she could be with David and talk with the surgeon or any other doctors who might come to check on his progress.

A day and a half after his surgery, David suffered a setback. He had a grand mal seizure. It was seen and reported by the nurse who was caring for him. His surgeon explained to Barb that seizures were not unusual when the body is recovering from the shock of major surgery. But to be safe, he called in a pediatric neurologist for a consultation. This new development worried me. Would the neurologist discover more problems to deal with? Hadn't we all been through enough? We were both present when the neurologist and two resident doctors came to examine David. They huddled around his bed like a solemn conclave, talking among themselves. I watched as the neurologist tested David's reflexes and movements. He let David fall backward from a sitting position. He moved a bright-colored toy back and forth in front of his eyes. He moved the same toy swiftly toward David's face, stopping just before his nose. As I watched all of this, and as I tried to read the doctors' faces for some clue as to what they were thinking, I grew scared inside. There seemed something foreboding in the way that one test lead them to try another, then another. What if he had suffered some neurological damage? How bad could it be?

The neurologist ordered a CAT scan of David's head. The films showed that David had suffered an "edema" or swelling of the brain, which he attributed to the episode of respiratory failure, the lack of oxygen. However, he reassured us that the swelling and the seizure activity were temporary. They would disappear after a few days of medication. In the meantime, they would keep a close eye on him.

Day by day, David improved—with some minor setbacks. An early attempt to wean him from the respirator had failed. However, samplings of his blood were showing slow increases in oxygen level. The brain swelling had gone down. The incision in his chest was healing. Though he was not "out of the woods" yet, everything looked promising. Barb and I were hopeful.

His ten days of hospitalization were becoming an enormous strain on both of us, but especially on Barb, who spent most of her days and nights there alone. I would make the trip to the hospital each night after work and on my days off. On several occasions, friends or relatives drove up to spend some time with Barb. But for the most part, she was on her own, keeping vigil over David, bearing up under the emotional strain of his setbacks, and trying to communicate with doctors and nurses who used a jargon she often could not understand. On one occasion, she fired an angry outburst at a resident doctor who was speculating as to whether David's eyes were impaired. On two other occasions she broke down in front of me, swearing she could take no more of this. We had been living on the edge of anxiety. It was, especially for Barb, an exhausting routine set in a depressing environment. More than anything, we wanted to take our son home and resume our lives. The joy of childbirth and of parenting had become lost or faded under the tension of these fearful events. We both felt cheated.

Finally, the day arrived when we were told that we could take David home. We were overjoyed to leave the hospital and the frenzied existence behind, and to once again take on the normal roles of mother and father at home. We could start over and feel like a family again.

The doctors sent us home with two ongoing prescriptions for David: Digitalis, to keep his heart rate regular, and Phenobarbital, to control seizures. They couldn't be sure that a seizure would not occur, even though the brain swelling had gone down.

From the time we brought him home, David was a different child. He was very fussy and irritable. He wouldn't smile for us. He didn't even seem to look at us. It was very difficult to make him feel contented. He would no longer suck on his pacifier. In fact, he barely sucked on his bottle. We had to begin delivering all or part of his feedings through an oral syringe, as we did for his medications. This made for a long feeding process, but we were willing to do it. We wanted nothing more than to nourish him back to good health.

Two weeks later, David began to appear lethargic. His appetite was down, and he seemed to be less active in his body movements. When our pediatrician examined him, she recommended that he be seen by his cardiologist at the nearby children's hospital.

Upon examining him, the cardiologist recognized immediately that David was experiencing some congestive heart failure. He was tachycardic, meaning his heart rate was too high. Because the heart was not pumping efficiently, fluids had begun to build up in his liver and other internal organs. An adjustment in his Digitalis medication would be required to bring everything back into balance. Once again, David was admitted to the hospital. Having just healed from his last hospital stay, he now had to have some of his hair shaved and an IV inserted into his head again. He was wired to a heart monitor. They began administering a new dosage of Digitalis through the IV, along with Lasix to help him urinate the excess fluids from his body. The rest of the process was simply to wait for what they called "conversion", that is, the point at which his heart rate would drop to a normal, efficient pace. That occurred in the afternoon of his second day in the hospital. He let out a sneeze and his heart rate suddenly dropped down to a normal range. Though this surprised us, the cardiologist explained that sometimes a simple sneeze can bring about conversion.

After three days in the hospital we took him home. His fussiness continued, especially at night, when he would wake and cry. Barb and I took turns holding him and rocking him in a chair we kept in his room. Sometimes he was contented to be held and rocked, and would even fall asleep in our arms. But getting him from arms into crib was a dreadful task. We would hold our breath, hoping he wouldn't wake. Often he did, and the whole soothing process would start over again. Sometimes, too, the rocking did little or no good. On several occasions, we tried letting him cry himself to sleep. But this approach never worked. He would only scream and cry himself into a frenzy. By the time one of us went into his room to hold him, he would be warm and sweaty and hysterical. This brought on feelings of guilt and made us wonder if we were putting an undue strain on his heart.

In short, we were all losing sleep. These nightly vigils were taking a physical and emotional toll. We were tired. Sometimes even resentful. When the problem was described to doctors, they politely reminded us that David had a very rough start in this world and probably still needed time to recover. He was only three and a half months old. His pediatrician prescribed a change in formula, thinking perhaps his stomach was having difficulty handling the present one. But that did not help. Nothing helped. We simply continued going about this nightly routine and trying to endure.

David was now four months old. Several weeks had passed since his last hospitalization. One afternoon Barb placed him in his automatic swing. He always seemed to enjoy the motion of it, and it seemed to have a calming effect. But after several minutes of swinging, his body suddenly went rigid, with his head turned and his left arm raised. He was quiet and trance-like. We removed him from the swing and laid him on the living room carpet. He did not change. Not knowing what was wrong, we drove him immediately to the pediatrician's office. Upon seeing him, she instantly concluded that David was having a seizure. We had never actually seen David in a seizure before, so we did not know how to recognize one. Up to this point, his medications had apparently kept him seizure-free. But now he was literally in the grips of one. A small oxygen tank was brought into the treatment room. Barb held the oxygen mask over David's mouth while his doctor called the children's hospital. Within minutes Barb and I were driving him to the hospital with the oxygen on board. On the way, he came out of the seizure and began to cry. He was admitted to the hospital for tests and evaluation and possible adjustment of the anti-convulsive medications he was taking. A pediatric neurologist was called in for consultation. Over the past weeks and months Barb and I had been hopeful that David was recovering from the effects of the brain swelling episode that resulted from his respiratory failure. His doctors had referred to it as an "insult" to the brain and assured us that it was something from which most babies can bounce back. But the sight of his small body involved in seizure was terrifying, and it fostered new fears and doubts in my mind.

David remained in the hospital for two days, undergoing blood tests, an electroencephalogram and neurological exams. He was sent home with a new prescription and placed under the care of the consulting neurologist, who made an appointment for the three of us at his office the following Saturday.

I had to work that day, so I arranged to meet Barb and David at the doctor's office at our appointed time. It was a hot, sunny June afternoon, the day before Father's day. We met the doctor not in an examination room, but in his private office. He sat behind a large desk. Barb and I sat in front of it, side-by-side in a pair of office chairs. She was holding David in her arms. The doctor began by reviewing David's recent hospitalization, his seizures, and the medication strategy he was using to control them. Then he paused.

"What kinds of things do you see happening with your child's behavior?" he asked.

With that prompting, we began talking about our frustrations with David's fussiness, his crying at night, the difficulty of feeding him, the fact that he never seemed to look or smile at us, and other complaints.

Another pause.

"I don't think the two of you are facing the fact here."
"What do you mean? What fact?" I asked.
"The fact that your son has suffered irreversible brain damage."

His words had no edges, no sympathy, no feeling, but they had the penetrating quality of electrical current. I could feel a wave of shock and fear run through me, all other emotions suddenly draining from me. I was trembling inside. For a few seconds that seemed like minutes, all of us were silent. I couldn't turn and look at Barb.

"Brain damage?" Barb repeated the words, intoning a question.
"I'm afraid so. Apparently the result of anoxia that occurred during his episode of respiratory failure. Have you not been aware of this?"

The answer was no, we had not. Every doctor and professional we had spoken to referred to David's condition as a temporary "insult" to the brain. No one seemed to second-guess it. No one expressed any doubt that he would recover. No one ever said he was permanently brain-damaged. Now, here sits this neurologist telling us in a calm monotone that our child is ruined!

"How bad is it?" I asked. "What are we talking about?"
"It's relatively severe," he answered. "We're talking about a child with multiple handicaps."
Barb asked the next question — the one I was afraid to ask: "What kinds of handicaps?"
"Severe retardation. Cerebral palsy. He will probably never walk or speak or demonstrate consistent patterns of meaningful cognitive behavior. He will probably also exhibit growth failure. I'm afraid this child will not make you very happy."

Then he directed us to an examining room, where he showed us a high-intensity light gun. Because the skulls of newborns and infants are so translucent, he explained, they allow the penetration of light into the cranium. Damaged areas of the brain are more recessed from the skull, and therefore show up more brightly under the light emitted from the gun. He dimmed the room light and clicked on the gun, holding it over various areas of David's head. The light was penetrating in relatively large patches. As I looked on and listened to him pointing out in a clinical manner specific areas of damage, I felt sick inside. To hear the diagnosis was one thing, but to see it so starkly now under the light was quite another. Every hope, every dream I had for my son instantly dwindled into nothingness, like inflated balloons whose air stems are suddenly let go. Everything gone, flown. Nothing left inside me but this sick, scared feeling.

After the exam we returned to his office and sat down. We asked a few more questions. Barb asked for a long-term prognosis for David.

"What you must understand," he said, "is that there is no cure for your child's condition. The long-term picture is not very bright. Children such as David usually have many health problems that can shorten their lives. Many of them have a proneness toward upper respiratory problems, such as pneumonia. Many of them have a tendency to aspirate liquids or food or their own vomit. These things can be fatal. Most children with problems as serious as these die at a young age, roughly ten or thereabouts. David's health is compromised not only by his neurological condition, but also by his heart disease and growth failure. Do you have any other questions?"

If we did have any, we were too much in shock to think of them, too numb to ask them. He wrote us a prescription for pediatric valium to be given to David at bedtime. "Whether or not you use it is entirely up to you," he said. "But under the present circumstances you are both burning yourselves out by trying to accommodate him all hours of the night. The valium will help him to sleep through the night and allow you to get a good night's rest. And that's what all three of you need."

We walked out of the office and down the hallway in a daze. As we descended silently in the elevator, the physical sensation seemed to be the perfect metaphor for what was happening inside of me — a terrible sinking feeling. Barb and I did not speak a word to each other. We walked out of the building into the bright June sun, where everything seemed strange and remote to me, as though I had stepped from another world. I fumbled for the right key to unlock the door of Barb's car. She stooped in and fastened David into his car seat, then turned to face me, her lower lip quivering.

"Now what?" she asked.
I looked down at the ground, shaking my head, at a loss for words.
"I don't know," I replied.
For a few moments we stood in the parking lot, beside the car, and held each other, as though it were the only thing humanly possible left to do. And we cried.

The tears that welled up from inside of us were tears of despair, confusion and grief. Finally, we had been given a bottom-line diagnosis of David's problems. There was no longer any room for hope or confidence or pride or celebration. Any plans for his future were not merely postponed — they were canceled. One single incident, one medical crisis had suddenly wrought a lifetime of unyielding depredations. The news left both of us empty inside, uncertain of the future, and even somewhat scared of our own child.

We got into our cars and drove our separate ways. I had to return to work, although it was the last place I wanted to be right now. On the other hand, I didn't want to be at home either. If I had my way, I would have gone someplace where I could be alone, to think or to cry.

For the rest of the day nothing else occupied my mind except the bad news about our son. The neurologist's conversation played over and over again in my mind: "I don't think the two of you are facing the fact here." His words were like an accusation. Why hadn't we been given any facts to face, I wondered. How was it possible that, for all these months, doctors had either overlooked this diagnosis, or had been afraid to tell us, or had simply assumed that we already knew what we were dealing with?

I thought about the future and what it might hold, not only for David, but for Barb and me. No longer could I see myself, years down the road, playing outdoors or hiking with David, or perhaps teaching him woodworking. No longer could I picture the three of us doing something — anything — as a family. In fact, there no longer seemed to be a future: it had all been wiped out in a matter of minutes that afternoon. I could only see my son years from now, older and bigger, strapped limply into a wheelchair, drooling on himself, face contorted. It was a bleak and ugly picture. And it filled me with an anguishing, gut-wrenching revulsion.

Wouldn't it have been better for David to die before or during that surgery, I thought, instead of being allotted a life not worth living? In saving David's life, they also saved his death — a death we would have to look at each day, every time we held him, fed him, bathed him, changed him, picked him up in the morning or put him to bed at night. He was no longer the same child we brought into this world: that child died. In his place now was a child severely retarded and handicapped. I didn't know him. How could I orient myself to such a child? How could I be a father to him? And did I really *want* to be a father to him? The questions swarming in my head were unyielding, and I had no answers, only an uncontrollable fear.

I had known several families with disabled children. I began thinking of each of them now. All of those families seemed to be well-adjusted and relatively happy. But perhaps those parents were special people. Perhaps they had the "right stuff" to endure the heartbreak and go on living. Did Barb and I have that same stuff? I seriously doubted it.

We were alone, paralyzed and powerless. Life as we knew it, planned it, was now relinquished. We were forced to accept something far less than what we had hoped for and expected that day we walked down the aisle three years ago. Instead of sharing the joys of marriage and family, we had to face a grim reality. Our child would have none of the milestones that other children reach with great hoopla and celebration: no first words, no first steps, no normal schedule of childhood development. Those things in life that are meaningful, enjoyable, fascinating and inspiring were stolen from David.

The shock of David's diagnosis was like watching, with disbelief, the entire dream break apart in our hands while we stared silently at the pieces, knowing they will never fit together again. How could our marriage endure such an undermining loss of happiness and fulfillment? It required more than merely surviving. It required gathering our entire lives into the singular sad acceptance of tragedy. That meant redefining happiness in far lower terms than I could conceive. It meant having to remodel our lives, and all of the plans we had laid, to accommodate something we did not expect or want. Disappointment was too shallow a word to describe the impact of the neurologist's diagnosis. I was devastated.

I could easily tell that Barb shared most of these same feelings. I returned home that evening depressed and tired from the thoughts and anxieties that had been pulsing through me all afternoon. Barb and I sat and discussed our shock, our numbness, how we couldn't believe what we had heard that afternoon in the doctor's office, how dispassionate he was in the telling of it. Before going to bed that night, we decided to tell our parents and families on the following day.

When I awoke the next day, it was Sunday — Fathers' Day. I walked into the kitchen and found two cards on the breakfast table waiting to be opened. One was from Barb. The second one she had signed David's name to. On the front it depicted a well-meaning little boy telling his dad to relax on Fathers' Day and let him take care of the chores. On the inside, it showed the botched and cluttered results of his efforts. I read it and began to sob. Barb leaned over my chair and put her arms around me. In a tearful apology she said, "You know, they just don't make a Fathers' Day card to fit our circumstances."

We drove to my parents' house for a Fathers' Day visit. I was apprehensive about telling them the bad news. After all, they had brought eight healthy, normal children into this world and raised them in a loving, nurturing environment. I was bringing them a grandson who was anything but normal and healthy, and deep inside I was questioning my own ability to love him. Before I gathered the nerve to tell them, Barb broke the news first, beginning with, "Well, David had an appointment with a neurologist yesterday...", then went on to explain his diagnosis. Their faces dropped. They asked questions about his handicaps and the prognosis, and we answered them as best we could. Then my mother reached over and took David from Barb's arms and held him. For some reason I felt a sense of relief and reassurance. And I knew by their words and gestures that, although they were heartbroken by what we had told them, it didn't diminish their devotion toward their grandson. They would stand by us and support us.

From there we drove to Barb's parents' home. Again, Barb broke the news. Her parents and grandmother, too, were heartbroken — not only for David, but for Barb and me as well. We explained everything the neurologist had told us regarding the handicaps David had and the long-term prognosis. And they, too, showed their sympathy and support, reassuring us that we were all in this together.

Telling our families the bad news somehow lessened the tension we were feeling inside. In the coming days and weeks we told other relatives and friends. In doing so, and without realizing it, we were spreading a network of sympathy and support that we would depend on in the months and years ahead. Announcing that our child was brain-damaged was difficult and sometimes awkward. Most friends and family dealt with the news in a way that made us feel comfortable. But there were those with whom we felt uneasy in the telling of it, knowing they did not know how to react — what to say, what to ask, whether to offer their sympathies or to make a fuss over David as if he were a normal baby. From the beginning, and throughout David's life, we were always open in any discussion of him. We wanted everyone to know and understand David — and us. Even more importantly, we wanted him to be accepted.

By the end of June we were searching for a babysitter. Barb had gotten an extension of her pregnancy leave from the General Motors division where she worked, but that leave was soon to expire. We felt it was necessary for Barb to continue working because her insurance coverage was so good. By now, David had already accumulated over $30,000 in medical bills. The coordination of benefits between her insurer and mine covered every penny of it. With all of David's medical problems, we knew there would be more expenses down the road. And besides, Barb simply needed the change of environment, the mental therapy, the diversion that a daily work routine can offer. It would give back to her a part of her life that was normal, and would remain normal. After interviewing several women, we began to realize how difficult it was going to be to find someone willing to babysit a child with disabilities, a seizure disorder and other health problems. By the time Barb had returned to work, we had found a woman — the friend of a friend — who lived close by. But after two days of caring for David, she informed us that she no longer wanted the job. She was afraid. It seems a nurse friend of hers had cautioned her about the liabilities of caring for such a child. So, we were back to square one. In the following weeks we tried two other babysitters, but felt uneasy about their performance. Finally, we interviewed a woman who worked in a living facility for profoundly disabled children. Although the babysitting hours conflicted with her schedule, she had a sister who was interested in babysitting a child in her home. We arranged to meet her. She was married and had a four-year-old boy. Her manner with David was gentle. She seemed relaxed and unafraid of him. And so she became, for the next two years, David's daily caregiver and good friend. Over time it became obvious that she had bonded closely to David and cared deeply about him. Barb and I were relieved, in the midst of all that was happening in our lives, to have someone so kind and trustworthy to care for him.

In the meantime, we started David in a therapy program at the hospital. Since I had the day off every Thursday, I drove him to the hospital for his weekly session. I would sit on the floormat with the therapist and watch her work with David as she explained her methods. Her diagnosis and evaluation of his cerebral palsy and neurological condition added several new labels to the already long list of things wrong with our son. But at least the therapy was something active and positive we could do for him — as well as for ourselves, to make us feel a little less powerless.

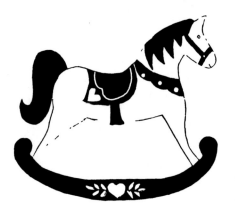

Chapter
Three

Barb and I were still very depressed. We were trying to close that enormous gap between expectation and disappointment, but finding it terribly difficult. Being forced to accept a family life that was far different than what we dreamed of and hoped for required us to make considerable adaptations in our day-to-day lives. Neither of us wanted to make such accommodations. But here was this child reminding us every day that we had no choice. Saddest of all was the unalterability of our situation, the painful awareness that there were no cures for David.

A deeply-felt despair penetrated every aspect of my life and cast a shadow over everything I did. At times I didn't feel quite like a father. True fathers have normal children, I thought. I didn't have a normal child and it seemed I was unable to handle that fact emotionally. Sometimes I felt angry at David for intruding into our lives and bringing all this turmoil. Though I certainly realized that David was blameless, he was nevertheless a visible scapegoat onto whom I could place my depression. On the other hand, these same hostile thoughts and feelings caused me pangs of guilt, and from the guilt sprang a sense of inadequacy as a father. The helplessness, the anger, the self-blame and the frustration all seemed to conspire against me in a way I could not control. I saw myself living life with my hands tied. I seriously began to wonder if I could ever feel happy again — ever.

I began working longer hours. That way, I could arrive home later, go through the motions of the evening routine, and not have as much time to think about my depression. In my spare time I threw myself into woodworking projects, one after another. Up to the time David was born, I had been working on a cradle that Barb and I had designed for him. It now lay in pieces in the basement, abandoned and incomplete. To finish it seemed pointless. Instead, I pursued other projects to keep myself busy. More than anything, I wanted some sense or illusion of normalcy. I wanted to shove all my depressing thoughts and feelings aside, or behind...or anywhere but inside me.

Over the months following David's diagnosis, our marriage became strained. We were both caught up in our own pain and anger. Each of us knew what the other was feeling, so what was the point of discussing it? We both needed to be comforted, but each of us was in too much emotional pain to comfort the other. Our conversations were not as long or engaging as they used to be. And when we did speak, the subjects were superficial, touching only the surface of things. We avoided opening our hearts and sharing those feelings of sadness and depression that were overshadowing our lives. We lost our intimacy. We isolated our "selves."

For both of us there was the added frustration of David's disposition, that is, his fussiness, his feeding difficulties, his obliviousness to everything around him. He never seemed to look at us. But the crying was the worst of it. Sometimes it was impossible to calm him. The pacifier no longer worked, since he had lost his sucking instinct. Often Barb and I would eat dinner in shifts, one of us holding David until the other was finished eating.

On one of those rare evenings when David was content enough to sit, propped up on the couch, we sat down at the dinner table together. We bowed our heads to say grace. Halfway through the prayer, Barb's voice stopped. I looked up and saw her crying. Then I began to cry. Nothing had been said. There was no provocation for the tears. Perhaps it was just the terrible irony of giving thanks for food on the table when the rest of our life was falling apart. Whatever the reason, we didn't explore it or discuss it. We simply dried our eyes and went about the business of eating.

Later that evening, I slipped on a jacket and went for a walk. As I walked, I thought about the painful events Barb and I were going through. I thought back to that day, three years ago, when we walked down the aisle together. We were so happy. Life was going to be so good. Little did we know how tough and miserable things could become in such a short time. I began to choke up again, but at the same time I felt anger rising in me. "Damn you!"

I whispered to God. "Look at what You've done to us! Why? Why?" Of course, there was no answer. I would ask that same question for years to come, and there would never be an answer.

David was our introduction to the unfairness of life. While the few friends of ours who had babies were looking at life with joy and enthusiasm, we faced a dismal, uncertain future. We often studied other babies David's age or older when we would see them at gatherings or public places. We sometimes wondered if the parents realized how lucky they were to have such whole and healthy children, or if they just accepted the fact as one of life's unquestionable certainties. Or did the sight of our own son awaken them to their blessings?

The first year of David's life was a precarious one. Every six to eight weeks we put him in the hospital for some illness — heart failure, seizures, pneumonia, viral infections. And each time, we wondered if he would make it. We had become very familiar with the hospital, the staff, and some of the medical procedures. We knew many nurses by first name. Weary of filling out my two-page insurance forms for every trip to the hospital or doctor's office, I made a set of photocopies to have ready at hand; all I had to fill in was the date and the reason for admission and/or the diagnosis.

It seemed we were moving between two different worlds: the hospital and the everyday world we were so familiar with and accustomed to. The world of the hospital was completely separate. Its environment was antiseptic and timeless. Inside its walls our daily routine was lost, given over to a chronology of medical procedures and events. The sounds, the smells, the flourescent lights, the furnishings all seemed conducive to an atmosphere of both boredom and anticipation. Finding ways to pass the time was often a ponderous labor, punctuated by a walk down a corridor, a trip to the restroom, a meal in the cafeteria, a conversation with a nurse or doctor. It was a world whose perpetuality left us weary, longing to be moving in that other world. Moreover, it was a world that forced us to open our eyes, to become painfully aware of sickness, suffering and misery among a population so undeserving of such affliction -- children. Before all of this, neither of us had realized how many sick children there are. But here they were, braving everything from mild illnesses and conditions to unendurable terminal diseases. Occasionally, we had the opportunity to speak to other parents in the hospital rooms, lounges or cafeteria, exchanging the stories of our children and their diagnoses. Sometimes these exchanges made our circumstances seem more fortunate; other times, less fortunate. But always such conversations were permeated by a vague but mutual recognition of a shared sense of pain.

David's sicknesses and recoveries were an emotional roller coaster for us. Even when he was "well" — if that word is appropriate —we worried about him. Over time, we developed a consciousness of how fragile his life was. Several times we even discussed his death, as though it were a near possibility. In an ironic kind of way, perhaps the anxiety of those sicknesses and medical emergencies is what helped to sustain us, by diverting our focus from our own depression toward the crisis at hand. Whenever David was in the hospital, I spent more time worrying about him than I did dwelling on my personal gloom. Barb would spend all days and some nights at the hospital, and I would drive back and forth after work each day. The busy-ness of these episodes, the discussions with doctors and nurses, and the pity we felt for our son were different kinds of mental activities. They allowed us to feel active and involved, instead of depressed and hopeless, and gave us other realities to space or separate us from the ones we were dealing with inside of ourselves.

Because of David's frequent cardiac episodes, his cardiologist offered to give him a brief examination, without charge, whenever we had fear or reason to suspect he might be in congestive heart failure. Since I was bringing David to the hospital once a week for therapy, I could conveniently stop in his office. I think he sensed the anxiety Barb and I were living under, and wanted to provide some relief. Whatever the reason, we were grateful and we accepted his offer.

Over time, we began emerging from the shock of our experience and gradually became more comfortable in our roles as parents of a disabled child. There were many factors that helped us along on this road to adjustment. Time was one of them. It seemed that with the passage of each month our emotional wounds were slowly healing. The impact of our personal disaster was lessening, and so was our numbness. The generous support of family and friends was another factor. They made clear their concern for David as well as for us. Their expressions of support, their presence in times of crisis, their offers of help all seemed generous mercies in sometimes merciless circumstances. But high on the list of those factors was the opportunity to meet other parents with similar experiences. On the recommendation of David's therapist, Barb and I attended a "pencil conference", an all-day educational seminar for parents of children with disabilities and for professionals who work with those children. It was, for us, an enlightening experience. We selected the workshops which we felt would be most pertinent to our situation. We learned a lot about being "special" parents, and we met other parents who were dealing with the same emotions and problems that Barb and I were. The keynote speaker was a child psychologist. In her address she described what happens to a mother and father when they find out their child is handicapped. "You grieve," she told the audience, "and your grief is perfectly normal and appropriate. You grieve because your child — the one you had hopes and dreams and plans for — has died. Therefore, a part of you has died. There is no greater loss. And that loss goes on living with you in the disabled child."

She went on to describe the stages of such grief, and how they parallel the stages described in Kubler-Ross's book, On Death and Dying. Barb and I were suddenly able to stand back and identify some of the emotions we had been experiencing over the past few months for what they really were. We had, indeed, been grieving. And we knew that grief has, somewhere, a point at which it diminishes and allows life to go on. "Understand your feelings," said the psychologist, "and you will own them. Once you own them, you can deal with them." We found a lot of reassurance in that thought. And we left the seminar that day feeling enlightened and even somewhat empowered by the things we learned and the people we had spoken to.

Perhaps what happened that day was like shock therapy. Barb and I attended this conference in a common interest. We read literature, we listened, we took notes. We somehow began to feel the need to be involved in our son's life in a more decisive way. A refreshing closeness came over us. I think the day was a catalyst in our long process of giving up that dreamed-of child we talked about during her pregnancy and reconciling with our real child in a way that would be positive and constructive. We still had our grief, our frustration, our fear and inner conflicts. But now we were finding something to balance those things -- as parents of a special child we were finding a sense of purpose.

We also joined a local support group called "Parents of Special Children", where we met a lot of other parents of mentally and physically disabled children. The sharing of emotions, frustrations, experiences and ideas was a tremendous benefit for Barb and me. Some of those parents had been successfully coping for years with the problems of raising a special child, and we took encouragement from that. If others could survive and endure — and find happiness in their roles — then perhaps we could, too. Among such people we found a unique kind of support that went beyond what family and close friends could offer — not to diminish their love and concern. But here were people who had been there, who had walked — and were walking — the path that Barb and I were set upon. Their support went beyond sympathy: it amounted to empathy and understanding, because they knew, because they were living the experience. We began to realize we were not alone.

As time passed, our lives seemed to be taking some kind of shape and balance again. David's fussy temperament began changing; he was able to calm himself for longer periods of time. We could prop him up on the sofa or in a chair, or in his automatic swing, and free ourselves to do other things around the house.

Barb's mother often came over to take care of him or to help out with household chores. My own parents and family were helping out, too, by babysitting or just dropping by to visit. In all, it was a welcome change of mood for Barb and I. We began getting out of the house more, sometimes taking David along, whether to visit family or friends or simply to go to the store. We began enjoying life again as husband and wife. We rediscovered laughter and intimacy, and found support in each other through an acknowledgment and understanding of our shared roles. Our problems were not going to go away. We knew that. But we were finding the mutual strength to cope with them. We were growing into this special kind of parenthood, and we were doing it with more confidence and less anxiety.

Meanwhile, David's therapy sessions were not netting any significant results. By now, a typical child would have been crawling or scooting, rolling over, and beginning to sit up. But David was doing none of these things. Instead, his body was floppy and he had poor head control. When he became fussy he hyper-extended his body, arching himself backward and becoming rigid. Furthermore, he was not focusing on or visually tracking moving objects, or trying to visually localize the source of sounds or voices. Worst of all, we hadn't seen a smile on his face since the days prior to his brain damage. But we kept up with the therapy, realizing that it would be a long road and that our expectations would have to be both limited and realistic.

We had a good rapport with the therapist. She was always happy to see David and seemed to genuinely enjoy working with him. She and the other staff people thought it was so wonderful to see a child brought in each week by his father — they said it was a rarity. That made me feel proud. And those weekly trips to therapy became something I looked forward to, driving in the car with my son and spending time with him in some purposeful way. Without realizing it, I was growing closer to David — in a way I had not thought possible because of his handicaps.

I began to find other activities that David and I could share together. On summer evenings, for example, I would sometimes take him out for a walk around the yard. We had an acre of land, so there was much to explore. I carried him around, checking on the progress of Barb's flower gardens and window boxes, or the growth of fruit on the fruit trees, or the grapes on the vines. I would talk to him as we walked, as though he could understand me. And I sensed that he absorbed something from these one-sided conversations -- something far beyond words or literal meaning. He was listening to my voice. He was contented with that.

One day Barb purchased a back-pack style child carrier to use for David when we were in places where a wheelchair or stroller would be cumbersome or too much baggage. A friend of ours who is skilled at sewing made a couple of adaptations on it to lend more support where David needed it. We often used it to carry him around in crowded public places, fairs and festivals, or the mall. And I sometimes used it to take David on short hikes on the trail along the river or in the woods behind my parents' house, where I spent so much time as a boy. He seemed to enjoy these little excursions in the outdoors. Perhaps part of that enjoyment was the experience of sights, sounds, even smells he was unacquainted with, but somehow perceived.

Another time Barb came home from shopping with a surprise for David -- and for me. It was a child passenger seat for my bicycle. I was concerned about how safe the seat would be for David, who was floppy and unable to sit up on his own. "We'll just use some Velcro straps to give him extra support," Barb insisted. "He'll be fine. And I think he'll enjoy it." So I assembled the seat and fastened it securely to my bicycle frame. We fastened David into the seat with the original seatbelt. Then Barb fashioned additional chest straps to hold him firmly upright against the back of the seat. Barb waved as she watched us ride down the driveway and out onto the road. I kept glancing back at David uneasily, worried that he might be frightened by this new experience of balance and open-aired motion. Sometimes his head would sway in an almost drunken fashion as we took a curve or a turn. But he sat quietly, seeming to be enthralled with the sensation of movement and the accompanying breeze. And I knew then that this was the first of many bike rides we would enjoy together.

Life is filled with moments that, either individually or collectively, move the heart and mind. Many of those moments go by unnoticed. But some are recognized for what they truly are: a milestone, a turning point, a mark in time. One such moment occurred for me on a Thursday morning. I had the day off. Barb had left for work. That afternoon I would be taking David to therapy. But for now, I sat at the breakfast table drinking a cup of coffee and holding him on my lap. It was winter. Through the sliding glass doors in the kitchen I was watching the snow falling gently on the trees and backyard, enjoying the beauty and quiet of it. Then I looked down at David, his innocent eyes glancing erratically about, as always. Suddenly, for no known reason, it dawned on me how far I had come from my own uncertainty about loving him, caring for him, being a father to him. I had made the necessary adjustments in daily life that his special needs demanded. More than that, I had come to accept him as he was, to acknowledge the loss he had blamelessly brought into our lives, and to move beyond it. But, most importantly, I had come to love him. As if the moment was revealing itself, I realized that David had made his way into my life and my heart. Inside of that realization was a feeling of gratitude. I lifted him up, pressed him against my chest and hugged him! That moment is still with me.

In July, 1979, Barb became pregnant again. Though I had appeared to be happy about the news, it only added to my anxiety. With David, we already had more than we could handle, I thought. And now another child? It seemed like too much too soon. And what if something went wrong with this new baby? But Barb was hopeful, even optimistic, and her outlook became contagious. I slowly came around to the idea that this just might be the best thing for all of us. Nevertheless, I worried off and on about the baby's health. But as the birth of our new baby drew closer, we looked forward to the event with the hope of experiencing the parental joy and fulfillment that had seemingly been stolen from us by the tragic circumstances surrounding David.

By March of 1980 Barb was in her eighth month of pregnancy. She had begun to notice swelling around her feet and ankles, so she made an appointment to visit our family doctor, who was also our obstetrician. When he listened to the baby's heartbeat, he became concerned. The heart rate was much too rapid, and he feared that her swelling could be a pre-toxic condition. He immediately prescribed bed rest in the hospital. By 6:30 p.m. the same day, Barb was admitted to the labor and delivery ward and attached to a fetal monitor. As the night wore on, the baby's heart rate increased. Barb and I were becoming concerned, and finally expressed that concern to the resident doctor on duty. We told him about the problems with our first child, and he understood the reasons for our uneasiness. He, too, was becoming apprehensive about our baby's escalating heart rate. He called to consult with our doctor, as well as with David's cardiologist. By 11:00 p.m. some quick decisions had to be made.

"Your baby's tachycardia (rapid heart rate) has shown no signs of letting up," said the doctor "It would be dangerous to allow it to go on. But the problem cannot be treated in-utero. In other words, we have to get the baby out and begin medicating it immediately."

He wanted our consent to authorize an emergency caesarian section. Faced with no alternative, we agreed. We were shocked and scared. The recent memories of all we had been through with David were flashing through our minds, making us brace ourselves for the worst. We could not believe this was happening — and happening so fast.

By 12:15 a.m. Barb was wheeled into surgery. They permitted me to go in with her, but because it was an emergency, and because something might be wrong, Barb and I agreed that it would be best for me to wait in a lobby close by. I sat and stood and walked off the minutes while my worst fears paraded through my mind. I prayed frantically, but was filled with an awful sense of foreboding. I did not want this child to be another David.

At 1:10 a.m. a nurse entered the room.

"Mr. Greenwald?"

"Yes," I answered.

"Congratulations. You have a baby girl," she said with a smile. "Six pounds, six and a half ounces. We're cleaning her up right now. You'll be able to see her in a few minutes."

I walked out to the hallway to stand near the doors of the delivery room. A transport team from the local children's hospital was standing by. Moments later, our doctor wheeled an isolette through the doors and stopped in front of me.

"Here's your daughter," he said, smiling.

I looked down at her. She seemed perfect in every respect.

"You can touch her, if you like," he said.

I reached my hand through one of the ports in the isolette and placed it on her tiny chest. I called her by the name we had chosen this time for a girl. "Katie," I said softly, "Hang in there, Katie." A few moments later, they whisked her away in an ambulance.

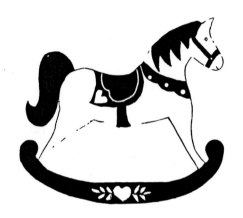

Chapter
Four

Katie's life began with a month-long stay in the neonatal unit. She was very sick, due mostly to her premature birth. David's cardiologist was able to stabilize her heart rate using the same medication that David was taking daily. Through this and other medications they were able to relieve a lot of the fluid that had built up inside her small body. Hence, in the 24 hours after her admission, her weight had dropped down to four pounds, seven ounces. She was on a respirator, unable to breathe on her own. She was diagnosed with Hyaline Membrane Disease, a common condition among premature infants. The Hyaline Membrane that covers the lungs at normal gestation is not completely formed, causing breathing difficulties. While Barb was still recovering in the hospital, I would drive to visit her after work, and then drive to the children's hospital to spend time with Katie, or vice-versa. On one occasion, I was in the entry area of the neonatal unit scrubbing my hands, preparing to "gown up" for my visit with Katie. A doctor poked his head around the door.

"Mr. Greenwald?" he asked.
"Yes," I answered.
"We just received word that your son is being brought by ambulance to Emergency. Apparently he's having breathing difficulty."
"Oh, God!"

I dried my hands and ran down to the Emergency receiving area. David's babysitter was just entering, carrying him in her arms, followed by an ambulance driver. She appeared shaken. I looked at David. He was crying, but otherwise seemed all right.

"What happened?" I asked.
"He just began coughing and couldn't stop," she answered. "He was crying and his color was changing and I was afraid he wasn't catching his breath. He finally settled down on the way here. I hope I did the right thing."

I reassured her and thanked her for taking the course of action she chose. David was brought to a triage room where doctors and nurses spent about half an hour examining him and taking his medical history. But nothing was found wrong with him. They speculated that perhaps the coughing was triggered by his own saliva. When they released him, the babysitter took him back home to allow me time for visits with Katie and Barb.

After a week, Barb was released from the hospital. For the next several weeks we spent much of our time together at the neonatal unit, where we were allowed to hold Katie and feed her. After several setbacks, including a ruptured lung from the respirator, Katie was weaned from the respirator and was breathing on her own. Within the thirty days she spent there she had gained weight, although she was still tiny, and was feeding very well — so well that we were able to bring her home. It was a happy day and a relief from the replay of those same anxieties we had been through with David.

Toward the end of Barb's pregnancy I had resolved to finish building the cradle I had begun for David. I had not completed it for him because of all the turmoil that overtook us after his birth. I could not find the will to complete it after his diagnosis because the project somehow, in my own mind, lost its symbolism and significance. Then, with Katie born prematurely and confined to the hospital for her first month, there was no time to pursue it. But now that she was home, I picked up the abandoned pieces and began the project anew, cutting, shaping, sanding and, finally, staining and finishing the wood. I built a music box into the bottom of the cradle. On the top of the mattress board I carved this inscription: Built with Love for Our Children. May, 1980. On the afternoon I finished it, Barb and I carried it up from the basement and placed it in Katie's bedroom. Then it occurred to me that it would only be proper to christen the cradle by laying David in it first, even though, despite his small size, he was too big now to use it.

I don't know what possessed me to finish the project so long after I had forsaken it. Perhaps it was a partial reconciling of the conflicting feelings I had experienced in fathering a disabled child.

Perhaps it was an acceptance. Perhaps it was simply a paternal inclination. Whatever the reason, I felt a certain pride and fulfillment that moment I lay our son in the cradle I had begun for him and finished for Katie. For me, it was more than a piece of furniture. It was an emblem.

From the very start, the differences between Katie and David were obvious. As Katie grew and developed, they became even more so. Katie could suck from a bottle, smile, follow objects with her eyes, hold toys in her hands, and express a curiosity about the world around her. In a way, it was like having our first "real" baby. All of those special moments that we had been deprived of with David were now being given back through Katie. But at the same time, Katie's normal developmental abilities made us more painfully aware of the severity of David's disabilities. As a result, we found ourselves sorting through a mixed bag of emotions, counting the blows as well as the blessings. We celebrated and treasured every milestone that Katie reached, but always with a self-consciousness of what David was and what he might have been.

When David was about fifteen months old, his therapist recommended that we have him thoroughly evaluated by a clinical psychologist. The idea seemed rather academic, since we already had a practical and realistic grasp of where David was developmentally. Nonetheless we followed through on the suggestion. The psychologist asked us a lot of questions about David's behavior. Then she ran through a battery of tests with him — very basic exercises such as reflexes, tactile sensations, focusing, visual tracking, noise response, motor movement and muscle control. As we sat there watching each procedure, we could see David failing terribly in most of the tests. Although his performance was not particularly shocking to Barb and I, it was nevertheless saddening. Here he was, being measured against the standards of function and development for normal children his age, to have his mental and physical disabilities defined in scores and numbers. The only numbers important to us were the ones appearing at the bottom of the evaluation report: "David is functioning at a 3- to 4-week age level."

Barb and I discovered that, for us, the emotions attached to having a disabled child — especially the grief and the anger — never really went away. We had a predisposition to such feelings. They were innate. They were part of the emotional turf that went along with being a special parent. They subsided for a while, only to resurface again, prompted by any kind of event, from a birthday, to a psychological report, to a seizure episode. Such things would cause us to dwell on the disparity between David and other children, and to feel sadness for what life holds for him. It was as though all the crises and depressing circumstances surrounding David's life were somehow fused together. When a new one came along it seemed to spark all of the previous ones and rekindle those feelings of grief, helplessness and frustration that overwhelmed us so many times before. If there was anything to be thankful for in this whole cyclical process, it was that there were reasonably long intervals between such episodes and events. Over time, this made our stress easier to cope with and allowed us to recognize the factors that induced it.

By now, I think Barb and I had, for the most part, passed beyond that self-pitying question, "Why us?" Now it was more a question of "Why him?" — why this innocent child? Why was he cheated in life? How does this square up, how does this reconcile with everything we know about a God who supposedly loves children? Why should his entitlement be any less than that of other children who come into the world? But, as always, such questions went unanswered. And as time passed, they were asked less frequently, not because they were irrelevant questions that did not deserve to be asked, but because the asking was often passionate, painful and frustrating. In such matters we ended up surrendering our sense of reason as a way of coping.

Although David was still very small and well below normal weight, he was showing some growth in length. He was also gradually losing some of his infantile features and becoming more "boyish" looking, especially in the face. As he outgrew his infant fashions, Barb replaced them with toddler clothes that seemed to make him look older. In a way, I didn't want to see this transition occur, because the bigger he grew and the older he looked, the more his disabilities were apparent to me and to everyone else. Out in public, people used to look at the little boy in our arms and often comment, "You've got a tired little baby there." But now there were more looks and less comments, as though people recognized there was something wrong with this child. I was never actually embarrassed by the stares, but I was always conscious of them. The day finally came when David was too old for the therapy program he had been enrolled in at the hospital. He was referred to another program at a local university, funded by a grant through the same hospital. Barb and I joked that we now had a son in college.

The ultimate "coming out of the closet" occurred when David began his new therapy program. One of the first recommendations the staff made was for a custom-designed wheelchair. They felt it would be very beneficial for David in terms of body positioning, visual perspective, feeding therapy and other areas — and would benefit us, as well. So we followed their recommendation and had a wheelchair/car seat built to accommodate his specific therapeutic needs. This became a kind of turning point in the way we presented David to the world. After all, when you stroll a child through a public place in a wheelchair, you are — like it or not — telling everyone you've got a disabled child. The sight creates a lot of visual interest -- head-turning and double-takes. But we learned to live with it. In fact, over time we became proud to take David out in his wheelchair and to address the curiosity of anyone who would ask about him. He was a special child, and that endowed us with a sense that we were special, too.

David's new therapy program involved some of the objectives of the previous one, but also established some new ones. There were several therapists who worked with him, all of whom were wonderful, dedicated people who seemed to show a genuine concern for David and a belief in the goals they were setting for him. It was a different environment from his previous program — more children, more therapy rooms and more therapeutic and adaptive equipment. Barb, along with Katie, took David to therapy sessions four days a week. By this time, she had quit her job to be at home with our children.

Along with David's small spurt of growth came the onset of more seizures, most of them small myoclonic seizures, consisting of sudden body jerks, sometimes accompanied by a turning and throwing back of his head. The frequency of them was disturbing — sometimes a hundred or more a day. He had been on two drugs — Phenobarbital and Dilantin — to control seizures. One of the side effects of the Dilantin was swelling of the gums. As a result, David's teeth, for the most part, had not come through; the few that did were almost buried in gum tissue. Barb and I were concerned about what kind of long-term problems this could cause for David, especially if he were to someday have the ability to chew food. His neurologist had been insistent on the use of Dilantin. We decided it was time to change not only his medications, but his neurologist as well. So we made an appointment with a pediatric neurologist on the staff of a large, renowned hospital. When we met him for the first time he tousled David's hair and spoke to him in a perfect Donald Duck voice. After examining David and putting him through some tests, he talked with Barb and I about David's problems, even showed us the results of the CAT scan he had ordered for David. It was the first time we had ever seen CAT scan films of the damaged areas of David's brain, even though David had previously had CAT scans. So here, at last, was a doctor who would share information with us, who would address our concerns, who would listen to what we wanted for our son. And what's more, he treated David with gentleness and compassion.

He prescribed new medications for David, explaining that there would be a weaning process and transition period required to get him off the Dilantin and on the new drug, called Depakene. Beyond that, there might also be a need for adjusting the dosage in the event that we saw any seizure activity.

We left the office feeling good about this new doctor, and about his strategy for controlling David's seizures. Within a month David's seizures had completely subsided, except for rare "breakthroughs." Shortly after, his gum tissue receded and his teeth finally came through. Now he looked even more boyish.

This had not been the first time Barb and I changed David's doctors. During his first twelve months of life, through crisis after crisis, we had dealt with many doctors and healthcare professionals, and we learned much along the way. We learned that these people are not infallible, that each of them brings a different personality and attitude to the profession, and that none of them knows our son like we do. We learned that most of them were good at hearing, but not always good at listening. We learned that many of them who serve small children with disabilities have little understanding of what the parents are going through. This is important to know because, after all, many of the child's problems impinge in a very direct way upon the parents. And we learned to ask questions and not to be intimidated by professional jargon. We had become consumers of medical services, and, as such, we had the right to select or reject the provider. What we wanted most from David's doctors was a willingness to share information in an open, understandable manner; a willingness to let Barb and me "call the shots" on important decisions, especially those regarding critical care; and a sense of compassion and respect for our son. These are qualities that doctors either do or do not have. When we found them lacking, we opted for a "personnel change", if possible. As parents, we recognized an obligation to speak for our son, who could not speak for himself, let alone understand all of the medical experiences he was being subjected to. Therefore, we learned to be bold when the situation called for it.

David's medications required monitoring to be sure that he was maintaining a therapeutic level in his body. This was done through blood tests. Every few months, we would take him to the outpatient lab at the hospital. Usually, a technician would come into the waiting room and carry David down the hallway into an exam room. As we sat waiting, we would hear David screaming from the prick of the needle. Sometimes they had to do this more than once, because he was a fast clotter — one of the effects of his heart disease. It tormented us to sit there and listen to our son crying out of pain and fear. After several such episodes, we decided that David would never go through this procedure alone again. From that time on, when a technician would approach us in the waiting room with arms extended and say,"I'm ready for David," I would simply stand and say, "I'll be going in with him." Then I would carry him to the exam room and hold him and talk to him during the blood-drawing process. Some technicians did not approve of my intrusion, but I never gave them the opportunity to have it any other way. I insisted on being there for my son and, although that may not have lessened his pain, it probably lessened his fear. It certainly lessened ours.

One of the new goals of David's therapy program was to teach him to eat from a spoon. David was about twenty months old and, up to now, we had been feeding him strained foods and cereals through an infant feeder, a kind of bottle with a large-hole nipple at one end and a collapsible bottom at the other. But since David would not suck the food through the nipple we would force it into his mouth a little at a time by applying pressure to the bottom of the bottle. Once the food was on his tongue he had to swallow it. But this was hardly the way for a twenty-month-old child to enjoy a meal! One therapist began working with David on spoon feeding by experimenting with the position of the spoon in his mouth and the proper placement of food to trigger closure of the mouth and a subsequent swallowing action. One evening when I arrived home from work, Barb announced that David would be eating that night's supper from a spoon. This was something I had to see to believe! She tied a bib around his neck, propped him up on her lap, and began feeding him one spoonful at a time from an electric warming dish. Every spoonful had to go in twice because it would run out his mouth. He fussed, and sometimes he would clamp down so hard on the spoon that there was nothing she could do but wait until he let go. After about an hour he finished the last spoonful. It was a long and messy procedure, but it was a beginning. We were pleased and proud, and we applauded our son all the way through his dinner. This was a significant milestone for David — one that we were doubtful he would ever reach, one that most children reach shortly after birth. But in caring for David, we learned to celebrate the insignificant — that is, the less remarkable aspects of development that go by unpraised or unnoticed by parents of other children. Therefore, whether it was an improvement in feeding, drinking, visual tracking or just learning to hold his head up and move it from side to side, we discovered in ourselves a certain pride and joy in David's achievements. That pride included a desire to share those achievements and demonstrate them for grandparents and family and friends.

However, for each of David's successes there was also a failure. In fact, there were more failures than successes. In those months beyond his diagnosis we sorted through the shards and pieces of our broken dream looking for something to salvage, to cling to, to hope for. We wanted to believe that, despite his multiple handicaps, there were still some basic skills and goals that David could achieve. Before realizing that David was severely brain-damaged, his surgeon and other doctors reassured us that infants and children have an amazing resilience, an ability to bounce back from brain insults. Therefore, even after his shocking diagnosis we continued to cling, in a hopeful way, to the notion that he just might bounce back -- at least partially -- and surprise us with the things he'd be able to do, the basic skills he would master. Such was the stuff of which stories were written and movies were made. We blindly held out hope because we wanted these things not only for ourselves, but for our son. We wanted his life to be better, somewhere in the near or distant future, than it was now.

Both of us -- but especially Barb -- worked with David, trying to reach him, to stimulate him, to elicit some response from him that would indicate we were connecting or communicating in some way. We would bounce him on our laps, tickle him, talk baby talk to him, sing to him and move his arms and legs. I would sometimes lift him high above my head or "roughhouse" with him on the living room carpet. We would move brightly-colored toys or objects across his midrange of vision to see if his eyes would follow them. We would use toys, bells, speakers or musical instruments to create sounds, hoping he would visually seek out the source of the noise.

With the help of his therapists we set some very limited, fundamental goals. At times David seemed to be approaching a level of achievement toward some of those goals, but with others we could find no consistency. Sometimes we wondered if we were only kidding ourselves by seeing success where there really was no consistent and reliable measure for it. And sometimes, too, David failed completely, leaving no doubt as to how realistic our expectations had been.

Such failures precipitated conflicting attitudes of determination and surrender for Barb and me. When we realized that standing or walking were not realistic goals for David, we changed the goal to crawling. We would work with him, trying to let him experience the sensation of bearing his own weight on his arms and knees. But he could not do it on his own, and it soon became obvious that the goal of crawling was not a realistic one. Perhaps scooting or rolling would become his method of locomotion. But again, over time we realized that these also were not going to come to fruition. David could not scoot or roll over. What's more, he demonstrated little or no interest in any kind of meaningful body movement.

With each failure we found ourselves having to lower our expectations. In this whole process of scrapping some goals and setting lesser ones we were learning the severity of our son's disabilities. At the outset, what we had to face was a frightening, and sometimes confusing, array of labels applied to him by doctors and therapists. Here is just a partial list of some of the terms they applied to David's cerebral palsy: "diffuse spasticity with muscle contractures", "primitive reflexes", "elevated muscle tone", "tight-fisted hands with bilateral cortical thumbs demonstrating no voluntary grasp", "strong asymmetrical tonic neck reflex", "bilateral hip flexor tightness", "adductor tightness", "neck hyperextension" and "quadraspastic". But those labels were medical terms that had only a vague reality. What brought them into sharp, clear-cut definition for us was David's failure to achieve so many of the goals we had set for him or to reach the normal stages of childhood development.

Those goals also represented something beyond their manifest purpose. They became fixed points in our hearts and minds -- metaphors for hope, for the vision of what our son's life could be. In that process of constant reassessment I don't know what was more painful for us -- the fact that some accomplishments simply were not going to happen for David, or our own resignation in the face of such fact: the act of giving up, and the nebulous sense of guilt and disappointment that accompanied it. Barb would sometimes question whether or not she was being aggressive enough, whether or not her methods were right, whether or not she was spending enough time working with him. But with me working and Barb caring for two children and both of us trying to maintain a household, it was impossible to allocate all of our time to constant therapy routines.

There were, however, some important goals that David did achieve. How much of that achievement can be credited to therapy, to evolvement and maturity, or to a combination of those factors is uncertain. What is certain is that those accomplishments were gratifying to Barb and me, as well as his teachers and therapists, in a heartfelt way.

For example, David developed a significant degree of head control. Immediately following his brain damage his neck muscles were unable to lift and support his head in a midline position. This ability is an important one because that midline position lends so much to a child's visual perspective, the awareness of his/her body and the environmental space that surrounds it. David's head was floppy, usually slumped downward toward his chest. When he did lift his head, it was only for a brief moment. Then it would roll back down to its passive position. But gradually, and with seeming willfulness, he was able to hold his head up for longer and longer intervals while sitting in his adaptive chair or lying on his belly. For reasons that had nothing to do with the obvious importance of this development David's new-found head control was exciting for us. Here was our son, plagued by so many disabilities, doing something -- and doing it apparently deliberately! It was wonderful.

Another of David's achievements probably evolved in no small way from his ability to control his head. He began, rather sporadically, to track moving objects across his field of vision, something he had not done previously. That is not to say he would track consistently. But over time there was a marked improvement in the frequency of his tracking, as well as the extension of it to the left and, especially, the right side. A noise-making toy or colorful object was sometimes enough to capture his visual interest and coax his eyes to follow its movement. Around age five he also began to demonstrate an effort to turn his head in the direction from which a sound was introduced -- in particular, our voices. The possibility that David was recognizing and identifying us through our voices was both thrilling and fulfilling. Sometimes Barb would hold him comfortably in a quiet room and make cooing sounds. At first, David seemed to show little interest. Then suddenly, one day he responded in kind by returning a cooing sound to Barb. From that time forward he would do this sporadically and not always with consistency. But it sparked our excitement, giving us hope that there was some kind of communication or, at least, acknowledgment going on, however rudimentary.

David also learned to calm himself when he became fussy or agitated, with little or no intervention from Barb or me. This was previously unimaginable. When David became fussy, the crying usually progressed from intermittent to constant, until he would work himself into a frenzy. One of us would have to hold him, rock him, gently pat him or perform some other calming technique until the crying would subside. And the incidents were frequent. But he seemed to gradually gain a greater degree of control over his fussy moods. He would still cry and complain, but for much briefer periods. This development was a great relief to us and made our lives less stressful.

Like other parents of disabled children, we sometimes felt jealous of typical children we saw in other families. Ironically, we also felt twinges of jealousy toward other children with disabilities not as severe as David's. Over time we came to know quite a number of other disabled children through David's therapy programs and through our support group. In our own thoughts we would compare David with these other children. We would note that many of them were able to walk, perform manual tasks, talk or communicate in some fashion, or demonstrate a variety of these and other skills. Almost none of them was as severely disabled, mentally or physically, as our son. This clear and visible fact made us sometimes perceive these other parents as being fortunate, having lesser disabilities and less heartache to deal with. We would fantasize about the opportunity to pick and choose which disabilities our son would have -- if he had to have them at all. At the very least I would have eliminated his retardation, leaving him with only his physical disabilities, but with the capacity to think in concrete and abstract terms, to learn, to understand, to converse and interact with us. For Barb and me this was the most frustrating and painful issue to cope with: our son was so severely retarded that we would never get to "know" him in the way that most parents know their children. We would always love him, yes. But he would, in many ways, always remain a stranger.

As Katie grew and became more verbal, she expressed a lot of curiosity about David, whom she referred to as "Deeda". I can't say whether her understanding of David's condition grew more out of our frequent explanations to her or simply from her experience of growing up with him. As a toddler, she often showed interest in playing with him, and a certain bewilderment at his inability to interact with her. Many times we tried to explain to her that David was "special", and therefore she was a "special" kind of sister, and that although he was unable to play at toys or games with her, he nevertheless loved her very much. We explained that David had disabilities that prevented him from doing the things that she did, but found that this was a difficult concept for a young child to grasp. At this age she herself often referred to David as having handicaps, but without a real knowledge of the impact and limitations they imposed on his life. Over time, she learned to be affectionate and gentle with him. She sometimes asked to hold him, and we would seat her at the corner of the couch and place David in her arms. (By this time, her physical size had already far exceeded his!) She would hold David awkwardly, stroke his hair, and talk to him in a motherly fashion: "Hi, Deeda. Are you looking at me? Are you looking at me, Deeda?" Other times she would sing one of her improvised songs to him.

But Katie also exhibited a normal sibling jealousy of David. His needs often required more time and attention from us than did hers, especially at particular parts of the day. Our expenditures of time, love and energy on the two children were often disproportionate — or at least sometimes seemed that way to Katie. When she felt neglected — if only in her own mind — it was nevertheless a reality to her that had to be addressed. Just as Katie had to grow into an understanding of her brother's special requirements, so we, too, had to learn that Katie's needs — physical, emotional and otherwise — were just as important as David's.

The burden of juggling the demands of the children fell largely on Barb, who had quit her job in order to be at home with them. Now with two children competing for her attention she had to devise ways of dividing time, or tending to both kids at the same time. Only in the evenings when I came home from work, or on my days off, did she get respite and assistance. I usually fed David his dinner, bathed him, medicated him and spent the better part of the evening holding him while reading or watching television. Oftentimes, I would cook the family meal also. Barb and I adjusted to sharing certain roles and wholly assuming others, and this helped us to balance the load and to cope. That is not to say we never had conflicts over day-to-day routines. We did. Sometimes one or both of us would feel overwhelmed or depressed by the burden that David placed upon us, and we would let it be known. But the next day, we picked up and carried on.

Caring for David was the same as caring for an infant: he was totally dependent, unable to do the most basic things -- like roll over or change position -- for himself. He was unable to communicate, unable to walk or crawl, unable to hold things in his hands, or feed himself, or toilet himself. As his spoon-feeding improved, we began giving him soft table foods like stews, pastas and vegetables, each of which had to be ground by hand to make them edible and digestible for him. In learning to eat from a spoon, he had achieved a skill which, had he been normal, would have relieved us of some work. Instead, it now created more work. What sometimes made David's care more burdensome, however, was the realization that this would never end, that David would always be infantile, and that we would always be doing everything for him. It was not that we viewed David through the prism of his disabilities. Rather, his disabilities began to define our relationship to him. Certainly, we could not have that playful, interactive relationship enjoyed by parents of typical children through the various stages of development. With David's development -- or lack thereof -- came the encroachment of distinct or implicit realities: there would be no games of peek-a-boo, no patty-cake, no hide-and-seek, or chasing through the house and yard; there would be no teaching him the alphabet or how to count to ten; there would be no mischievous episodes or toy-strewn rooms to clean up. And, worst of all, there would be none of the wonder, the discovery, the humor so often inherent in the perceptions and conversations of a child.

In the course of absorbing and dealing with such realities, the nature of our relationship to David was evolving from one of parents to one of caregivers. That is not to say we no longer cherished or fulfilled our roles as mother and father. Indeed, we continued to love and nurture this special child of ours in every way. But so many of our points of contact or connection with David revolved around his physical needs: feeding, diapering, bathing, clothing, positioning, transporting, therapy, or the things

61

he required for contentment. Our roles as caregivers became more pronounced as he reached the ages or stages when typical children take on such everyday tasks and responsibilities themselves. Such negative thoughts and depressions, however, did not last long. And the resentment they built faded quickly. We did the things we had to do because we loved him. The extra care he required became as routine as the normal care required by Katie.

In our minds David was, first and foremost, our son and Katie's brother. Among our families he was always thought of as grandchild and nephew. No one seemed to define him in terms of his disabilities. No one seemed to regard him as a broken person or thing. He was flesh and blood, human and wonderful. But among those who knew us less, or not at all, there were sometimes different perceptions of David or of us, his parents. Some looked upon him with pity or discreet curiosity. They felt sorry for us and said things like, "I could never handle having a child like this. I don't know how you do it." Well, we "did it" because we had no choice. This is what life had handed us, and we learned to live with it only because we had to, not because we wanted to, not because we had asked for a child like David.

Other lines we heard occasionally were, "You must have been chosen by God," or "He must be a gift from God." Although well-meaning, such ideas seemed to defy basic theology and our own perceptions of God. At my angriest, I saw David more as a sign of God's neglect or abandonment, or even cruelty, than as a gift. I could look at the present-day world and, seeing a lot of misery and injustice, easily conclude that most of these things were inflicted on man by man. But this — this child — was God's fault. And the idea that a disabled child is a gift from God seemed utterly naive, a contradiction against the God I thought I knew.

At age three David became eligible for enrollment in the school for mentally/physically disabled children that serves our county. After visiting one of the "Early Childhood" classrooms and speaking with teachers, we were impressed with their program and decided to register David. He began attending in the summer of 1982. In a classroom of seven children he was the smallest child. In fact, he was the smallest child in the school. Two of the children in his class were able to walk, several could crawl, and the others, like David, required wheelchairs and adaptive equipment. The classroom staff consisted of a teacher, an assistant teacher and two aides. The curriculum was very activity-oriented, including music, art, gym, swimming, speech therapy, and physical and occupational therapy. Barb and I felt good about the choice we had made. David was now being exposed to a lot of new activities as well as a wider social environment. There were new sights, new sounds and new discoveries for him. His teachers were wonderfully supportive and enthusiastic. They thought nothing of taking the children on field trips all over town — no small task when you consider the logistics: bundling them up, packing their special lunches, strapping some into wheelchairs, getting them on and off the bus, strolling the wheelchairs during the walks, taking time out to feed them lunch, medicating some of them, diapering, and generally looking after each child. It would have been far easier to spend every day in the classroom, but these teachers went the extra mile to offer something more to their students. Barb began to volunteer both in the classroom and on field trips. I also went along on some of the field trips that coincided with my days off: the zoo, the county fair, the amusement park and Christmas Land to name a few. We discovered how much these children enjoyed being exposed to new environments and experiences — and how much fun we could have with them.

We were grateful to have such creative and imaginative people in David's life, as well as in ours. Over time we developed a good rapport with all of his teachers. Many of them seemed to take a special liking to him. Sometimes, during summer break, one or two would come to our home to visit him. While Barb was in the hospital for several days after delivering our third child, he spent overnights at each of his two teachers' homes. David's teachers and therapists were important people in his life because they so willingly spent their time and care on him. They were important people in our lives, too, because by their commitment they inspired in us a greater love and acceptance of our son. They shared their knowledge and skills with us. Their supportiveness helped us not only to cope, but to realize that we could cope happily, that our lives could include him and still maintain some sense of normalcy.

On a typical school day Barb would wake David up at 7:00 a.m. She would diaper him, dress him, wash his face, medicate him, and feed him his cup of formula through an oral syringe. By 8:30 the school bus stopped at the end of our driveway. She would carry him on board and fasten him into a special car seat installed just for him. The other passengers -- also children and adults with disabilities -- seemed to take a liking toward David, as well as demonstrate a curiosity about this "baby" who rode along with them each day.

David's class began at 9:00 with a routine called "morning circle". The children were arranged in a circle in their chairs, wheelchairs or adaptive seats. The teachers sat in the middle of the circle and led the children in songs of greeting. Sometimes the children were given noisemakers or instruments to play along. Morning circle also included other activities, as well, such as storytelling, playing simple games and listening to recordings. The rest of the school day was given to learning activities with a therapeutic emphasis: art, music, gym, along with physical, occupational and speech therapy. With such a small class and adequate staff, there was a lot of one-on-one attention given to each child. Even lunchtime was a form of therapy. Some children were learning to spoon-feed themselves; some, like David, were learning to tolerate being spoon-fed, trying different tastes and textures in foods, and learning to drink from a cup. The school cafeteria offered the options of regular meals, or chopped or pureed preparations. Barb usually chose to send a lunch in with David so she could control his menu and provide him with foods he liked.

After lunch there were more activities, followed by a "nap time", during which the classroom lights were turned off and the children were laid on cots to rest or sleep. At the end of the school day the children were diapered, jacketed and placed on their respective buses bound for home. David's bus would arrive at the end of our driveway about 3:30 p.m. Barb would board the bus, remove David from his car seat and carry him into the house. She usually sat down with him for a while, holding him on her lap and talking to him. Then she would lay him on a blanket on the floor, or prop him up on the couch, or place him in his bed, and let him listen to music until I had his dinner ready. Such was a typical day in David's life. Though it may seem routine -- and it was -- it provided structure and, perhaps, predictability and anticipation in his daily living. It was also beneficial to Barb, because she was now free to spend a larger part of the day on activities of her own choosing. She no longer had to transport David to and from therapy. She and Katie could come and go without having to load and unload a wheelchair from the car. In the beginning of the school year she missed having David with her. But in a short time she realized that his new schedule and new surroundings were better for both of them, and she enjoyed the respite.

Feeding therapy was one of the programs we had established for David during his IEP (individualized education plan) proceedings. IEP was the process by which we and all of the teaching and therapy staff involved with David got together at the beginning of the school year and outlined specific goals for David and steps for achieving them and what services he would require. By now David was finally spoon-feeding, but was often unrelaxed and temperamental during a meal. His head often turned toward the left side, the side he tended to favor, instead of a midline position. And he had little jaw control, which meant that he tended to suck and swallow his food. Here is what his occupational therapist wrote after initial feeding observations and evaluation:

David sits in a Tumble Form feeder seat which is strapped into a desk chair. A wedge and additional foam pieces are placed behind his head to bring the head into slight flexion. The head and trunk are fully supported as his own control is poor. Increased muscle tone is apparent throughout his body. When David becomes upset, the muscle tone increases and the upper extremities pull back into a flexion pattern.

A Mothercare spoon and a small Tupperware midget cup (with cutout space for nose) are used as utensils. David's mother sends in his food; it is a consistency between ground and pureed, with some texture to it. David is fed from the front with full jaw control provided by the feeder, as his own jaw control is poor. David was observed to close his lips on the spoon part of the tine. A moderate tongue thrust was observed; David will push food out of his mouth if not given jaw control. David sucks his food rather than chewing. No tongue lateralization is noted; occasional biting on the spoon is observed.

At times David may refuse to open his mouth or open it with the tongue tip up. This makes it difficult for the feeder to insert the spoon. The tongue elevation seems to be due to the increased muscle tone and overflow patterns. David also tries to turn his head while feeding, but the feeder tends to keep it in midline through the use of external jaw control. David appears hypersensitive to touch, but his reactions vary from day to day. David is able to take a few sips at a time from a small cup, but will lose some of the liquid. Jaw control is needed while he is drinking.

The occupational therapist designed various components of a feeding program for David that involved positioning, relaxation and calming techniques, spooning techniques and cup drinking techniques, all spelled out in step-by-step fashion. As can be imagined, lunchtime was generally messy for David and some of the other children and required a considerable cleanup effort afterward.

There were other areas of concern that became part of David's IEP programs throughout his enrollment in the county school: increased muscle tone; muscle contractures and decreased range of motion in his movements; poor head control; scoliosis; visual tracking from side to side as well as up and down; and general awareness of his environment. These concerns and variations on them became the basis of our IEP conferences and of the objectives and strategies set forth by teachers and therapists. At the end of his first school year, an annual assessment report stated the following:

David has made gains in improving head control and visual tracking skills this year. Neck extension has improved to where David is able to raise his head while in a prone position without using reflexive action and often maintains the position for about 10-15 seconds at a time. Neck flexor muscles still remain weak and little active neck flexion is observed.

David will track objects in a horizontal direction about 70-75% of the time. He will watch objects moving to the right more readily than objects moving to the left, and seems to prefer certain objects over others. He will occasionally watch an object move in an upward direction for a short period of time, but soon looks away. Occasionally he will follow an object across his visual midline, but usually only follows from the midline outward. However, David appears to be much more visually aware and alert than at the beginning of the year.

Therapy sessions have also concentrated on improving weight-bearing on the upper extremity. (That is, raising his upper torso with his forearms while lying on his stomach.) At this time David is doing minimal weight-bearing but usually does not fuss when put in the position or given the proprioceptive input.

Static positioning splints were made for David this year because his hands were becoming tight and there was a slight tendency toward deformity. At this time David is wearing the splints for one to two hour intervals, and occasionally will tolerate wearing the splints during a nap. The splints are designed to maintain range of motion in the wrist, fingers and thumbs.

Most of these were ongoing concerns that spanned David's four years at this school. It also seemed that David might have a vision problem. Barb, in describing David's visual abilities, always used the analogy of a camera without film. In other words, David was able to see objects and movement with his eyes, but was unable to mentally process what he was seeing. But over time it seemed that he was seeing clearly only at close range, based on his tracking response to visual stimuli.

Early in 1983 when David was almost four years old, we had an Evoked Response Audiometry test performed on him. It was prescribed by his school therapist. This was done while David was asleep. The electrodes for an electroencephalogram were attached to his head to monitor the brain-wave response to sounds coming through headphones. Since David was unable to signify whether or not he heard a given sound, this was the only accurate way to measure his hearing ability. The test results indicated some hearing loss in his left ear. These sight and hearing deficits were not shocking to Barb and me, but they were nonetheless saddening and discouraging. This posed further obstacles to our son's ability to achieve, to learn, to grow in awareness.

By the end of his last school year, these were some of the evaluations and observations made by his therapists:

David is a very involved cerebral palsy child with mental retardation, seizure disorder and optic atrophy... In evaluating range of motion and muscle function, all passive movements were measured, as David has minimal active movement.

David is able to lift his head with the tone in his neck extensors but does not have any co-contracture in the flexors. David uses his neck extensors so much that he has contratures in extension to the left. He does some visual tracking, but no other gross or fine motor skills are noted. He has very flared ribs and is still a belly breather. In supine he is at the mercy of gravity pulling his shoulders down against the surface. In prone, he is still weight-bearing on his cheek with his head turned to the side... In sitting with support, David just sinks into the support being given or arches back into extension. David does not have a positive support reaction when placed in the upright position depending totally on the support of the therapist.

In the area of Communication/Language, these observations were made:

David is generally non-verbal but will make cooing sounds occasionally with familiar people. He is generally quiet when content and whines or cries when upset or distressed.

David displays inconsistent responses to sounds and voices. He is visually impaired, but it is thought that he can see objects/pictures within 10-12 inches from his face and has demonstrated appropriate eye gazing to pictures. Minimal attainment of visually tracking an object.

Barb communicated with David's teachers on a daily basis by writing in a notebook that traveled back and forth with him each day. This communication became very beneficial to us and to his teachers. One of his teachers wrote, "I look forward to your letters. You are the only one who writes to me. Everyone else writes notes about colds, medications, information or instructions. Your notes are always personal." Following are a few samplings of letters from David's teachers.

9-2-83

Barb & Bob,
    Hi. Guess what David gave us today in morning circle? A long smile!! We were singing about hand cream, rubbing his hands--such a sweet smile!!
    Also today we propped him up with a pillow in front of a mirror with 2 pictures on it. He kept moving his head, looking at both pictures very intently. So he's done two really neat new things for us today. We are very proud.

Penny & Kathy

7-8-84

Barb & Bob,
    David seemed fine today. He wasn't fussy at all. I worked him real hard and he didn't seem to mind. He was watching everything that was going on in the room. He seems to be so much more aware of things.
    David ate so well for me today, he was a little pig. I was able to apply some jaw control without him fussing. I almost forgot--he drank a whole glass of juice today.
    He looks so cute in his sailor outfit and tennis shoes.
    Thank you all for coming with us to the zoo yesterday. I think it is great when families participate in the school program. Please send towel and swimsuit for David. Swimming tomorrow.

Penny & Kathy

On the last day of school in 1985, David's teacher said goodbye to him. He would no longer be enrolled in her class. She sent along this lovely note with David.

6-14-85

The Greenwalds:

This is a sad day for me. It will be very strange not to have David in our room. Over the past three years, Kathy and I have grown to love David and your family. I feel lucky to have shared so many times with all of you. David is lucky to have two of the most caring parents any child could ask for. We will miss the daily letters; no one else writes us as often as you do, Barb. I'll come over to your new house again to see all the changes (the before and after). Good luck with the house and with Bob finding a new job.

Thank you for everything.

Love,
Penny

4-9-86

Dear Barb,

David had a seizure at 11:15 a.m. for 15 seconds while he became rigid, according to Marion who was holding him at the time. As I am looking at him, he seems alert and okay.

A few minutes ago (1:45 p.m.) David had a second seizure of about the same intensity and length of time. He appears to be very relaxed and about to fall asleep.

I hope he has no more today.

Lu

These are only a few samples of correspondence culled from nine notebooks filled over four years. Often the exchanges between Barb and David's teachers included things going on outside of school, their lives, their personal interests, what they did on the weekend, etc. Through Barb's notes they learned more about David and about our family. Through their notes we learned more about his teachers, as well as each day's activities at school, what new experiences David may have had on a given day and how he responded to them. They reported everything from bowel movements (David had chronic bouts with constipation.), to seizures to mood descriptions, to his progress in a particular learning activity or goal, to new foods or new activities they tried on David. This daily exchange of information kept all of us well-informed and, over time, developed a special friendship with his teachers that still exists today. They also sent home with David many "certificates of award" over the years. They were granted for a whole array of activities and achievements: "most improved head control"; "best BM!"; "best feeding session"; "best swimming session"; "first laugh"; "first smile" or any smile. His smiles were very few and far between. Barb and I were never fully convinced that they were real and deliberate because they usually appeared and then disappeared so quickly. We often thought that they could have been the result of sporadic movement of his facial muscles, that he did not even realize he was smiling.

But one Sunday morning he gave us no doubt. The evening before, we had attended the wedding and reception of David's teacher. It was a backyard affair with a live band and dancing around the swimming pool. In addition to many teachers and school staffers, she invited her students and their families. A number of teachers took David in their arms and waltzed him around. He seemed to enjoy it. The following morning after breakfast, we had him seated on the sofa when suddenly Barb called me out of the kitchen. "Bob, come out here quick!" I ran into the living room thinking that David had had a seizure or something. But when I looked, there was David grinning from ear to ear. "Can you believe this?" Barb asked. We knelt closely to him and stared intently, smiling and laughing with joy as we beheld this long, sustained smile accompanied by a moan-like laughter. We were in awe. We had never seen anything like this from David. "Quick, get the camera!" Barb said. When I returned to the room with the camera, David gave us enough time to snap a couple of shots and then that wonderful smile was gone, never to be seen again except on film. But it was one of those fine, rare moments that will always stay with us.

In his new school environment David was also exposed to a population of children who, like him, were prone to sickness. He caught his share of colds, flus and viruses — conditions that are adverse for even a normal child, but, for David, could lead to pneumonia and become life-threatening. Whenever possible, we treated his illnesses at home. Our family physician was very understanding about our desire to keep David out of the hospital. He worked with us by prescribing care and medications we could administer ourselves. Many were the times we set up a mist tent over his crib. Many were the times we immersed him in a tub of cool water to bring down a fever that had him crying hysterically. And many were the times we wondered, without verbally acknowledging it, whether he would recover from an episode of sickness.

Once, when David had a flu-like virus, he was feverish, crying hysterically, and unable to keep down food or liquids. Even his appearance attested to the fact that he was terribly sick. All day long Barb struggled to get food and liquids into him, but without success. He was even vomiting up his antibiotic and seizure medications. By evening, Barb, too, was coming down with the flu. The next day, I stayed home from work to take care of Barb and David and to watch over Katie. By now David was badly dehydrated. His lips were cracked and the inside of his mouth was dry. In a last-ditch effort to keep him out of the hospital, I began giving him fruit juice, drop by drop, through an oral syringe. I found that by giving him small increments like this he was able to keep it down, even though he gagged and cried throughout the procedure. It was a slow process, but I kept at it all day at thirty-to-forty-minute intervals. By evening I had gotten a large amount of liquid into him. It was working. He had become rehydrated and was wetting his diaper. The fever was declining. His crying had subsided. Barb and I, though exhausted, were relieved that he had made it through another worrisome crisis. By managing David's sickness at home instead of placing him in the hospital we were able to provide more comfort for him and be in control of his care and treatment. Although such episodes always boosted our confidence in our abilities to provide the kind of care that was best for our son, we never deluded ourselves or gambled on how severe a crisis we could handle ourselves. The hospital could well be the only proper place for David in some future sickness, and we could willingly accept that. We both knew that this would not be the last episode. There would be other crises somewhere down the road. It was just that way with David.

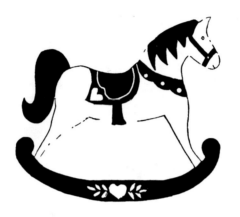

Chapter
Five

In the summer of 1983, Barb became pregnant again. It was a pregnancy we had planned. Although Katie was a wonderful sister to David, we felt that a "normal" brother or sister, with whom she could interact more playfully, would be a terrific benefit to her — and to us. Katie had begun to mimic some of the behaviors she had seen of other mentally/physically disabled children at David's university program and, later, at his school classroom. This bewildered us at times. Barb found it more disturbing than I did; yet I admit to wondering if her imitative behavior was symptomatic of something going on in her head — a feeling of being less loved, perhaps, or less tended to than her brother. Did she think the mimicking would draw more attention and affection? In the area of peer socialization, Katie was mingling and interacting more with children who had a variety of physical and mental disabilities than she was with non-disabled children. This was probably both good and bad: good in the sense that she was developing a first-hand understanding of and compassion for special children, but bad in the sense that she was often among kids who did not demand a higher level of play and social behavior. But this was not the sole reason — or even the main reason — for having another child. Quite simply, Barb and I wanted another. And how much David influenced that decision, or what factors came to bear upon it, we never tried to analyze. We were just happy and hopeful about this pregnancy.

On April 12, 1984, Steven was born. His birth was by scheduled caesarian section. Having stood in on the surgery, I was able to see him enter the world, an experience I had missed at Katie's birth. I even took a few pictures! It was a wonderful and joyful moment for Barb and me. "A baby boy in good health," was the pronouncement of the attending doctors, who had monitored closely the progress of Barb's pregnancy over the past nine months.

Two days later, on a Sunday morning, I dressed David and Katie in their nicest outfits and drove them to the hospital to visit Mom and to meet their new brother. Unfortunately, Steven had jaundice and had to be kept under the flourescent lights in the nursery until his bilirubin count came down. Katie, age four, showed a lot of excitement over the new baby, wishing she could hold him, and verbally demonstrating her big-sister affection for him. David, of course, was oblivious, unable to understand who or what this naked little bundle of life was, let alone what an important event had just occurred in his family. Yet it was terribly important to us that David be included in such moments. We held the conviction that, however limited his perception, however inattentive his disposition, however restricted his ability to express or react, his inclusion in family events was important. It was good for him and good for us. It bonded us more closely as a family and it endowed us with a deeper understanding and love for this little boy who seemed to live in his own world.

That morning, as I held David and we all stood staring through the nursery window at baby Steven, I found myself contemplating the immeasurable contrasts between these two children, as I had done four years ago when Katie was born. At present, our two sons were equals: infantile and totally dependent. But in the months and years to come Steven would clearly, visibly outdistance his brother in every aspect of growth and development. He would smile, laugh, and learn a language with which to communicate and share. He would crawl, stand, fall, then go on to conquer gravity with those first tottering steps. He would throw a ball, ride a bicycle, scrape his elbows and knees, and examine the world around him with an insatiable curiosity. In pondering all of this, I could not decide which was the greater wonder: that Steven would routinely grow through these common, yet miraculous, stages of life, or that David never would. It is a paradox that remains with me — and with Barb — even to this day.

Steven was the first and only of our children that we were able to bring home directly from the hospital. This worry-free birth experience was something new for us — and we enjoyed it. No trips back and forth to other hospitals, neonatal or intensive care units, as in the past. This time, we simply bundled up our new baby and brought him home. Now a family of five, our lives would become even busier than they already were. They would also become even happier.

Steven's first perceptions of David were much like Katie's had been — a curiosity and wonder toward this child who sat and did nothing, who did not speak or look at him. When Steven grew to the point where he could stand, he would often pull himself up beside the couch where David sat propped with pillows and pat him, or tug at his hand or foot. This always annoyed David and he let it be known by crying loudly. But Steven, like Katie, grew toward at least a fundamental understanding that his brother was "special." He, too, made trips with Barb and Katie to David's classroom and to other places where he met more children like his brother. At every opportunity we tried to enlighten him as to why David was different from him, why he was "special,"and why that made Steven a "special" kind of brother. Eventually, when Steven was big enough, we allowed him to hold David on his lap while sitting in a cushioned chair or on the couch. As he would look on, talking to him and patting him ("Gently," we would remind him), the protective, big-brother look on his face became obvious. There was a kind of benign irony in this: that Steven, like Katie before him, was assuming the attitude and, to a limited extent, the responsibility of an older sibling, even though he was less than half David's age.

However, Steven's interest in his brother was not without its mischievous moments. At such times we realized he still had a long way to go in understanding that David was a fragile human being — not a toy or plaything. On one occasion, he crawled up on the couch and stood up — on David's head! On another, he dropped several coins into David's mouth as he lay reclined. Fortunately, Barb heard David choking, saw some coins in Steven's hand, and realized immediately what had happened. She quickly turned David upside-down and out came the money. In another episode, Steven stuffed a small piece of snack food down into David's ear, requiring a trip to the emergency room to have it extracted. Each of these acts was innocent enough. Steven intended no harm to his brother. But the fact remained that David had been unintentionally endangered by his younger brother, who did not fully understand or appreciate the hazards that his curious, inquisitive behavior could cause. In time, he would come to that realization. But until then, we had to closely monitor his activities around David.

Both Katie and Steven learned to accept their brother as easily as they learned to accept each other. As they reached various levels of maturity we gave them more opportunities to share in his care and to do things with him. Steven, for example, sometimes pushed him up and down the driveway in a stroller. Katie learned to diaper him and dress him. As a show-and-tell project for kindergarten, she brought David into her classroom and, with Barb's help, talked to her classmates about David's mental and physical disabilities. She sat beaming, holding her brother in the middle of a circle of curious children, proud not only of him, but of herself. And we were equally as proud of her. Both Katie and Steven were assimilating an experience that most children never get. What was wonderful about it was not only their acceptance of it, but their desire to share it with others.

But it was also good that Katie and Steven could not understand or ponder the deeper implications of David's condition: how limited his life was; how trapped his soul was in a body and brain that did not work. Such sorrow is the domain of parents. Only a mother and father can appreciate the pain brought on by seeing in their disabled child their own dreams broken. Only Barb and I could reflect upon the tragedy of David's life and the sorrow it had brought to ours. Only we could fathom the enormous loss, the fact that David could not participate in the joys, the rhythms, the magic of life as typical children do. With the passage of time those feelings became less frequent. Our life with David was happy. We loved him. We were proud of him. Nevertheless, when thoughts of his misfortune would occasionally return and occupy our minds they brought with them a brief but stinging sadness.

Oftentimes I would stare at David when he was sitting or lying on the couch, with his music filling the still air of an afternoon or evening. Sometimes his eyes would have a distant, faraway look; other times they would seem alert, as though he were somehow seeing the music. "What does he hear?" I would ask myself, "What does this music mean to him? Is it a confused, yet pure, sensation? An experience of pleasure to the ear and brain? Does he sense a structure in melody and rhythm? Or is it a mere backdrop of his consciousness?" But those questions were merely spinoffs of the deeper questions that came to mind again and again: "What goes on inside that little head? How does he perceive the world around him? Can he formulate any kind of concrete or abstract thought within the narrow limits of his intellectual ability? With no concept of size and distance or time and space, with no ability to impose order on the thousands of sensory impressions that bombarded him every day, was he living in a world unexplained, an appalling darkness in which any attempt to process or understand could be simply a blind leap, and every shape and color was perhaps without substance or significance?"

Without the ability to speak or understand language, he could never communicate his feelings and desires, other than by the most infantile method – crying. Each of us uses words not only to communicate, but to think. We think in words. Words are, for everyone, the tool for establishing a human frame of reference by which we integrate ourselves into our physical and social environment. Words are the means by which we catalogue information, store memories, and attach meaning to people, events and things. Without words, it seems, experience cannot be interpreted or preserved. But David had no words. He could observe all he wanted to, but he could not distinguish objects by name, or describe or analyze his surroundings. Words, for him, were meaningless sounds that offered no connection to his closed world. Whatever went on inside that little head must have been as basic and elementary as etchings on a cave wall scrawled by primitive tribesmen, like simple stick drawings — not quite a language — depicting fundamental needs and desires. David's needs and wants seemed plain and simple — food and drink, a bath, a fresh diaper, the pleasure of music and of being held. He could not describe a "happiest day" in his life. He could not dream of new toys, new places, new experiences. And when such things came his way, I doubt that he held them in his memory, as most children do.

This was the mystery of David, a deeply perplexing one. Barb and I came to understand that disability creates a world of its own -- one that contains us, but only arbitrarily includes us. Along with loving and accepting him came the frustration of not really knowing him. That is not to say that he had no personality. He did. But it was not comprised of the sum of traits and qualities developed through interaction with people and with his environment. Nothing of his personality was formed through the kind of learning experience by which typical children assimilate and analyze the characteristics and values of their parents and culture. David's personality was more defined in terms of his passive responses to people and stimuli around him. In other words, he was his own person. We learned his likes and dislikes through everyday experience and discovered a reliable degree of predictability in his responses. We knew how to make him content, even "happy" sometimes. And we also learned the art of reading and gauging those often subtle responses. But it was only in this limited sense that we knew David. More than anything I wanted to get inside his head, to see the world as he saw it, to know how his mind wandered and wondered, to find, perhaps, some new thing that would please him or give him enjoyment. I wanted to reorder his small universe. If I had the power to give him something more than my love, it would have been language, perception, and a child's fascination, among many other things.

Along with these musings I also wondered often about the quality of David's life. Was he happy — or at least content? It was hard to believe that he could be, living in such a restrictive little world circumscribed by the boundaries of his disabilities. Yet the measure of happiness is relevant to personal experience. There are, for each of us, some good, joyful, or enriching experiences that we will never know; therefore, not knowing them, we do not require them in order to be happy. Perhaps it was this way for David. Perhaps, not knowing any other life, he found this life good. Perhaps his life and our love were enough. Barb and I wanted to think so. The sadness we sometimes felt for him might well have been inappropriate, having no relevance to his disposition.

Always at these moments when I would sit and stare at my son, I could not help but note what a handsome little boy he was. He had such a full head of hair and large blue eyes that seemed to me the emblem of his innocence. His clothes always complemented his good looks. Clothes tended to last David a long time. He was unable to dirty them, tear them or wear them out like a typical child. And because he suffered severe growth failure, he would take years to outgrow his clothing. Barb and I often joked that David took better care of his clothes than any child we knew!

But beneath his clothing was a body visibly frail, delicate and poorly developed. To see it for the first time was a shock for some people. At age eight, David weighed only fourteen and a half pounds and measured about thirty-one inches in length. He had no buttocks. His legs were simply like two small spindles extending from his torso. They were so skinny that his knees appeared to be knobbed. His arms, likewise, were small and scrawny. And his chest was sunken to the point where every rib was visible. His limbs were often dispositioned by muscle contractures, the result of cerebral palsy. This naked little body may have set others aghast, but it was the body his mother and I had come to love: the body we soaped, rinsed, and held close in the shower; the body whose diaper we changed again and again; the body we dressed and undressed daily; the body we sometimes stared at with sadness and wonder — wonder that he had survived this far, wonder about how many more years he could survive, given the odds his doctors had offered. Looking back, the question of how long David would live was always in my head during the early years of his life. Because he had such a difficult first year, Barb and I feared from the beginning that we might not have him for long. Indeed, there were times when we thought that death might be the best thing for

David because his life seemed like a prison. And perhaps our lives would be better, too. After all, he did place a lot of limitations on us as a family. There were places we could not go and activities we could not do with David along. And yet, having David along was important to us.

The idea that his death might be best for all of us -- including David -- was one that evoked feelings of fear and guilt. In other words, could it happen because I thought it? Was I really wishing for his death? If so, what kind of a father was I? All of these questions and the main issue they surrounded held the potential for much internal anguish and conflict. We loved this child. We knew that his death would be emotionally devastating for us. Yet we also recognized the freedom it could bring us. We could become a "typical family". Life would be easier. We would be relieved of the daily chores that David's care required, along with the stress and emotional turmoil. And for David it would mean heavenly peace and joy. But always hovering over these reflections and musings were the essential questions: "Are we being honest with ourselves? Are we being honest and unselfish toward David's best interests?" These ambivalent feelings could not seem to be completely resolved for Barb and I. In our hearts and minds the idea of losing our son scared us. Inasmuch as we sometimes fantasized about how much simpler life would be without him, the fact was we truly could not imagine life without him. We had assimilated our son. He had become us, a defining part of every aspect of our lives.

However, with each of his succeeding birthdays, both our speculation and anxiety about losing him grew less and less. His health seemed to stabilize. We had not had to hospitalize him for years now. And so that somber knowledge that David, in all probability, would not live a long, full life became buried in the backs of our minds, seldom contemplated. Not that we denied the idea of his death, but we began to regard it as something to occur in the far distant future. Now, at age eight, we considered that perhaps he had many more years ahead of him, as long as we continued to provide good care for him. We were soon to find out how wrong we were.

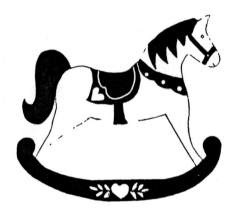

Chapter
Six

During the month of August each year, David had his summer break from school. August, 1987 was no different. He had been home from school for two weeks when, one day, we noticed an increase in his fussiness. We found nothing wrong with him and decided that perhaps it was just the boredom and inactivity of being away from his classroom that made him irritable. The following day he developed a cough, so Barb started him on Bactrim, an antibiotic we kept on hand for David's illnesses. Late the next night, however, he vomited. Barb heard him over the nursery monitor she kept at our bedside. She woke me and we went to his room. He had thrown up on his pillow. Fortunately, we had learned a long time ago to position David on his side when sleeping so that, unable to turn himself, he would not aspirate his own vomit. We laid him on the carpet and cleaned him off while he cried. She rocked him for awhile until he calmed himself, then placed him back in his crib with a fresh pillow. We went back to bed. Barb turned up the monitor's volume so she could listen in on David more closely. He slept soundly the rest of the night.

The next day, Thursday, I had finished work early and was home by mid-afternoon. When I entered the living room, I saw David seated in his adaptive chair on the couch, Barb next to him. He did not look well. His skin was pale, and his lips and extremities looked darker. He was feverish. Even his breathing did not seem right. Barb suspected he might be having cardiac problems. She said that she had made an emergency appointment to take him to the doctor's office. Shortly after, my mother arrived to babysit Katie and Steven. As Barb and I were getting ready to leave, David suddenly tried to sneeze, but could not muster enough breath to do so. This concerned us even more, especially when we noticed the worried look on my mother's face.

In his office, the doctor listened to David's heartbeat and respirations and concluded that a chest x-ray was in order. After examining the x-ray films he turned to show them to us.

"David has bilateral pneumonia. You can see the congested areas here and here," he pointed. "I know how you feel about

87

putting him in the hospital, but this is rather serious. I'm sure they can do more for him there than the two of you can do for him at home."

That old feeling of worry...or fear...or panic came over me. It had been years since he was last hospitalized. I looked at David, suddenly seeing or sensing how sick he was. Barb and I looked at each other and nodded our assent to the doctor's recommendation. He left the room to phone in his orders to the hospital.

We stopped at home so that Barb could pack some things for David and for herself. She would stay at the hospital with him. It seemed the best way to ensure that David's needs were properly met. After all, he was unable to communicate. And no one on the hospital staff would know the small, but important, things about caring for him: how to feed him, how he liked to be held, how to position him in bed, how to calm him when he became fussy. Sometimes, when David was ill, discontented, or simply wanting attention he would cry and fuss, hyperextending his body and working himself into a frenzy that he could not seem to bring under control. Barb could be at his bedside to soothe him and give comfort when he required it.

After being admitted to the hospital, David was placed in a crib in a room. We discussed his history and his current sickness with the resident physician on duty. We also discussed our wishes that, in the event that David's condition became worse, he not be put on a respirator or put through any kind of painful, invasive procedure. In his lifetime David had been through many hospitalizations and an awful lot of "heroic", but painful and sometimes risky, measures to save his life or pull him through a sickness. Because we loved him and felt an enormous compassion for him, we wanted to restrict any unwarranted treatment that would cause him more fear, confusion, and prolonged suffering.

Examining David, the resident physician noted his congestion, the pallor of his skin, and some swelling in his feet. He prescribed an antibiotic and Lasix, a drug that relieves the buildup of fluids in the body and stimulates urination. He also ordered an IV, a catheter, a heart/respiratory monitor, and periodic breathing from an aerosol mask.

I stayed with Barb at David's bedside until about 9:00, then left for home. While driving, I had the time and silence to think about all that had transpired, and about our conversation with the doctor. I became worried and scared. David had been through so many sicknesses, but for some reason it occurred to me that this could possibly be his last, that he might not pull through this one. I had no solid reason for thinking this — only that he was sicker than he had been for a long time.

I found it difficult to sleep that night. So did Barb and David. Barb rested on an uncomfortable cot next to David's bed. He fussed every time he had to breathe through the aerosol mask and every time a nurse disturbed his rest to take his temperature and other vital signs during the night.

On Friday, he showed little change. Two other doctors were called in for consultations — his cardiologist and an infectious disease specialist. They decided to pursue the present course and give the antibiotic more time to "kick in". The fever had left David, but now his body temperature was too low. They placed an electric water-heated blanket under his bed sheets to bring it back up.

Barb stayed by David's bed all day Friday. She was exhausted from the previous night's lack of sleep and from stress. When I called her again late in the afternoon I encouraged her to go home for the night and get some good, sound sleep. She could leave specific instructions with the nurses as to how David should b held, positioned and cared for. "Go on home." I insisted, "I'll sto₁ and spend some time with him after work." And so she did.

When I arrived at the hospital that afternoon I found David in an uncomfortable position in his bed. He was crying and perspiring. I carefully picked him up, mindful of all the tubes and wires attached to him, and held him in my lap. I talked to him and gently patted his chest. He settled down after a few minutes and sat calmly in my arms. He looked tired and worn out. I wished there was something I could do to suddenly make him well again. But, like most of his other sicknesses, this one was a waiting game, one in which we prayed for small mercies, one in which we longed to hear words like "progress" or "improvement" rolling from the tongues of doctors or nurses. We hated seeing David so sick and miserable. It filled us with pity. It made us feel helpless and out of control. Hadn't life dealt him enough misfortune, let alone this?

As I sat in the room and held him, I talked to him, telling him he would be getting better soon and returning home, and this whole ordeal would be over. "Just hang in there, pal," I said. After a while I laid him back down in the crib and positioned him comfortably. I stood there for a few minutes watching him to see if he was going to fuss, but he didn't. He was tired. And so I left the hospital and went home.

The next morning Barb arrived early at the hospital. She found David crying and somewhat agitated, even a little feistier than he had been. When she picked him up and held him, he calmed down immediately. As she sat in a chair holding him, she observed that he seemed more rested, more alert than he'd been in days. His breathing was a little less shallow. One of his doctors confirmed her observations. He called for another chest x-ray. The x-ray indicated some slight improvement in the right lung, while the left was still largely involved with pneumonia. But at least there had been some improvement — enough to give Barb a sense of relief and a big emotional boost. She decided to try giving David some fruit juice through an oral syringe; it had been days since he had taken any liquids by mouth. He took it eagerly. More elation! Barb called me at work to tell me the good news. When I heard it, I, too, was relieved. The worry and fear that had preoccupied me for the last two days was suddenly lightened. He was getting better. He was going to pull through! As Barb and I talked, we began speculating about when we could take him home.

A woman friend of Barb's came to the hospital to visit her and David. They passed the afternoon in conversation, taking turns holding him. This constant attention seemed to improve David's mood and his level of alertness. For Barb, it broke up the monotony of those long vigils in the hospital room.

I didn't get to see David that day. Since Barb was spending the day and night with him, I went directly home after work to be with Katie and Steven. Katie had made a gift for David — a sort of pillow made from a white handkerchief stuffed with cotton. Included with it was a home-made card with a crayon drawing depicting him in a hospital bed. She also scrawled a get-well message on it.

The following day, a Sunday, I got out of bed early and went to work —something I rarely have to do on a Sunday. But the store at which I had been working had come under new ownership. Today would be the grand opening. There was much to do in preparation for the anticipated onslaught of customers. At the hospital, Barb rose early, too. She wanted to go down to the cafeteria for a quick breakfast and be back at the room by the time the doctors were making their rounds.

When she returned, she found David awake and perspiring. He was less alert this morning. His color was pale; his hands and feet were mottled. When she lifted him to change his position she heard him gasp. Then the alarm on his heart/respiratory monitor went off. When a nurse looked in the window of David's room, Barb waved her in. She checked the connections of the monitor; they were fine. The alarm had gone off several times in the past two days for no apparent reason. Then Barb told the nurse about David's gasping episode, asking her if it could have been a seizure. She did not know, but she listened to David's heart and took his blood pressure. His blood pressure was elevated. She called in a resident doctor on duty. After examining David he ordered another chest x-ray, blood gases reading, and more frequent application of the aerosol mask.

A while later he returned to the room with the head nurse. In a sort of bumbling, awkward way he told Barb that although the x-ray showed more improvement, David had taken a turn for the worse. His blood pressure was up, certain blood gas levels were dropping, and his internal organs were backing up with body fluids — congestive heart failure.

"He's serious enough that we may have to move him to intensive care," the doctor said.

"Oh, I don't want to do that to him unless it's really necessary," Barb replied. "What would they do for him there that you're not already doing for him here?"

"I don't know. They might possibly put him on a respirator. But I don't know if he would be a good candidate for that kind of treatment. Let me go confer with the doctors in intensive care, and I'll get right back to you."

From the doorway of the room she watched the resident walk down the hallway. As she turned, she saw the elevator doors open at the other end of the hallway. Our family doctor stepped out. Barb ran down the hall to catch him and to tell him how sick David was and about the possibility of moving him to intensive care. She broke down and cried. As they walked toward the nurses' station, they noticed the small conclave of David's doctors talking among themselves.

"Let me talk to them and find out what's going on and what our options are," he said to Barb.

Barb returned to the room, where she stood beside David's bed and pondered the seriousness of the situation. Moments later, our family doctor came into the room and stood at the foot of his bed.

"The situation is bad," he said. "David has gotten much sicker. We could move him into intensive care."

"Have we done everything we can do for him in this room?"

"Yes, but I don't know that intensive care is the answer. In ICU the doctors would recommend putting him on a respirator.

But the doctors I just spoke with said they feel that David is so small and so sick that it would require a surgical procedure to hook him up to it. Surgery and anesthesia would be very risky. I know how you and Bob feel about pursuing a course like this. It's very invasive and would put David through more pain. Besides, there are no guarantees that this would work, especially in view of his present condition. It might only prolong his misery."

"Isn't there anything else we can do ... some other medication?" Barb asked desperately.

There was a short, almost ominous, pause.

"Barb, David is dying," he said gently.

His words confirmed what Barb had almost known, but was unable to admit to herself. Hearing the words from him directly and unambiguously gave her the strength to accept the fact, and to change her strategy from one of keeping him alive to one of making his death as comfortable as possible.

"Alright," she said, holding back her tears, "then I want to handle this the right way."

"What do you want?" he asked.

"I need a phone to call Bob and some other family members. I'd like a room without a hospital bed or monitor or any other equipment — a place where Bob and I can privately spend whatever time is left with David."

He left to make the arrangements Barb had requested.

It was 9:00 a.m. I had already been at work for two hours. I had thought about David during the morning, wondering if his doctor might give us a projected release date today. Then I received Barb's phone call.

"Hello."

"Bob?"

"Hi! How are you? How's David this morning?"

"Bob, can you get down here right away?"

Her voice was breaking. I could feel a sudden bolt of fear flashing through me.

"Honey, what's the matter?"

There was a brief pause, as though she was having difficulty bringing the words to her mouth.

"We're losing him," she answered, and began to cry.

I was in shock. "Barb, what happened? He was doing so well yesterday!"

"I know. I can't believe it either. But when I came back from breakfast this morning and found him awake, I thought he was uncomfortable because he was perspiring. So, I lifted him to change his position, and he let out a gasp, as though he were struggling for air. His color looked bad, too. They took more x-rays and saw a little more improvement in his lungs, but the rest of his internal organs are backing up with fluid. He's in congestive heart failure."

"Oh God, Barb! Isn't there anything they can do?" I asked, my own voice shaking now.

"They talked about putting him on a respirator, but said they would have to do a surgical procedure to hook him up to it. The doctor said he knows how we feel about such aggressive measures and he really thinks that it would put David through a lot of pain and would probably only prolong his misery. He said David is terribly sick. " Barb was trying to force out the words through her sobs. "He said David is dying."

And with those words all the hope I had inside me suddenly vanished. There was no asking whether there might be some mistake; whether, perhaps, the doctors might not have looked at this from every angle; whether there was some yet-unthought-of possibility, some card left unturned. Our son was dying. The words had a terrible finality to them. This was the reality we had pushed far back into our minds years ago. Suddenly, that reality was now re-emerging with a cruel, stunning impact.

"Oh, Barb, I can't believe this!" I said.

"I know," she answered. "Will you come down here right away? They think David could linger for three to four hours, so they're going to give us a private room with a couple of rocking chairs, so we can spend whatever time is left with him."

"O.K., Honey. I'm leaving right now. Bye."

I hung up the phone and walked over to another employee, who had asked about David earlier that morning. I had a terrible lump in my throat.

"I have to go to the hospital," I said, barely getting the words out.

"Is there a problem with your son?" he asked with concern.

"He's slipping away." I forced out the words and broke into sobs.

"Come on," he said, "I'll drive you there."

I tried to assure him that it wasn't necessary for him to drive me, but he was insistent. And perhaps he was right. I was upset and distracted. During the twenty-minute ride to the hospital he tried nervously to make irrelevant conversation, but I was too absorbed in the shock of what was happening. When we arrived at the hospital I thanked him, hopped out of the car, and jogged over to the entrance.

I emerged from the elevator on the sixth floor. Down the hallway I could see Barb standing at the nurses' station talking to one of the nurses. As I was approaching, she turned to face me. Our eyes locked together, as though recognizing each other's pain. When I reached her, we embraced and cried.

Since the nursing staff was unable to provide the kind of non-patient room Barb had requested, we had to make do with the room David had spent the last few days in. They drew the curtains over the window looking out onto the hallway and brought in two rocking chairs. They also brought us a pitcher of ice water and offered to get anything else we would like. The head nurse spent a little time with us to answer our questions and explain how David would expire. His breathing, she said, would become more and more shallow, his heart rate would slacken, and he might make an occasional gasping sound. Then Barb asked the question I was asking in my own mind: "Will he be in any pain?"

"No," she answered. "It will be like falling into a sleep. He won't experience pain or struggle. His internal organs are shutting down. He's so sick and his body is so weak that it is yielding to the process of the pneumonia and heart failure."

We stood over David's bed. He lay there with the aerosol mask on his face. We removed it; then we removed the electrodes of the heart/respiratory monitor. The nurse removed the I.V. from his wrist; then the urinary catheter. She began to put a fresh diaper on him when Barb interrupted: "I'll do that." As I watched Barb wrap the diaper around his small loins, I understood why she had insisted on doing so. It was the last time she would change his diaper. This everyday parental chore was suddenly elevated to a loving, caring expression. It was her last participation in one of those seemingly insignificant daily rituals that somehow bond a mother and child.

Throughout the process of being "disconnected" from all of the apparatuses, David fussed weakly. Now he relaxed in Barb's arms. The nurse left the room. We moved the rocking chairs side-by-side and sat down. As Barb rocked him gently, we stroked him and talked to him. We studied his face: the eyes, the lips, the nose, the ears, the wonderful head of hair. And there was an intensity to our observations, a self-conscious effort to take it all in, a desperate desire to memorize each and every one of his physical characteristics, as though we had not done so in these eight and a half years. We both remarked with tearful pride how handsome he was.

Then Barb handed him to me. She excused herself to go to the restroom. I continued to rock him and talk to him, stroking his face and hair. His eyes were half open, half closed. I wanted so badly to know that he was hearing my voice and feeling comforted. Then I noticed his breathing was becoming shallower, the rise and fall of his belly growing less pronounced. After several minutes his lips suddenly pursed and he gasped. I could feel the rush of fear or adrenaline pumping through me. "It can't be happening now," I thought. "The doctor said he would probably hold out for several hours. What's taking Barb so long?" He gasped again. "Please, David, don't do this," I pleaded. "Stay with us a little longer." I placed my hand on his chest to feel his heartbeat. He had always had a distinctive, pounding beat, due to his cardiac condition. Now the beat was very light and slow. I kept my hand there, feeling as helpless as him. I wanted Barb to walk through that door right now!

David gasped again — this time twice in a row, his small chest heaving slightly. I cradled him up higher, closer to my face. I told him I loved him, and watched helplessly as his life ebbed away. His eyes were closed and his breathing was now imperceptible. Minutes later I could no longer feel his heartbeat beneath my hand. At that moment, it occurred to me that I had witnessed my son entering the world and now leaving it. And in both I felt a profound sense of privilege. I laid my head against his chest and cried.

In the following minutes my mind flashed back through some of the many events that delineated his frail life: the diagnoses, the grueling surgery, the medical crises and illnesses. This small boy had suffered greatly and unfairly. Yet he also achieved some things on his own terms. How young he was, I thought to myself. How heroic.

Shortly after, Barb entered the room. She walked over to my chair and stood beside us, placing her hand on David's head. She must have seen the tears in my eyes or the look on my face.

"What is it?" she asked.
"I think he's gone," I said.
"Oh no!" she begged. "Please, not already!"
"I don't feel his heartbeat," I said.

With that, Barb took him from my arms, sat down in the other chair, and slipped her hand into David's hospital gown, letting it rest on his chest. I watched her face change, her lips quiver, her head bow lower until I could no longer see her face, but could hear her crying. I leaned over to put my arm around her, not only to comfort her, but to draw comfort from her. We both talked to David, telling him we loved him, that we would miss him. Then we fell silent, the only human sound in the room coming from our breath and our sniffling. Under the soft hum of the flourescent lights, we sat quietly for a while, laying our hands on him, touching and stroking him.

The head nurse peeked around the edge of the door to see if we needed anything. I told her that I thought David had expired. She bent over us and placed her stethoscope on David's chest for perhaps a half-minute. There was a seemingly long silence while we waited for her word. But without looking up, without saying a word, she simply nodded her head in affirmation. When she stood up straight she said softly, "You can stay in here with him if you like. Take as much time as you want. Just let one of the nurses know when you are ready to leave, and we'll take him."

"Take him?" Barb asked.
"Down to the morgue — only until he can be picked up by the funeral home you choose," she said, leaving the room.

I cannot describe the pain brought on by the thought of being permanently separated from our son. I cannot find words equal to the depth of grief we were feeling at that moment. Our hearts were truly broken. How could we let go of this child born out of our love; this child we had nurtured and cared for like a baby throughout his lifetime; this child we had seen through so many crises? As we stared at his lifeless body, we hugged each other and cried again.

"I wasn't there for him," Barb sobbed. "I wanted to be with him when he died, but I wasn't."

I knew that she would feel badly for not having been with David at the moment of his death. She explained that she was walking back from the restroom when she ran into a close friend whom she had called earlier that morning. She had tried to comfort Barb as they stood in the hallway talking; meanwhile, David was taking his last breaths.

"Barb," I said, "you didn't know he was going to die so soon. We both expected him to last for hours. Don't blame yourself. At least one of us was here with him. Besides, you've been right at his side for days here in this room. He knew that, and that's what's important."

She began rocking him in the chair beside me and patting his little bottom as she had done a thousand times when he was alive.

Two more very close friends, one of them David's godmother, arrived at the hospital hoping to see David, not knowing he had already died. Barb placed David in my arms and went out into the hallway to meet them and to break the news. A moment later she poked her head inside the door.

"Do you mind if they come in to see him?" she asked.
"No, I don't mind," I answered.

They entered the room, both of them crying, and walked over to an unoccupied bed where I was now sitting with David. They kissed him and touched him. Watching them do so without any hesitation or reservation gave me a kind of comfort, an affirmation that our son had truly been loved by others. They were sharing our grief now, as they had early on in David's life.

"Bob, we have to make arrangements." Barb said.
"Arrangements for what?" I asked.
"We have to choose a funeral home."
"Now?"
"Yes. I'm not going to have our son laying in some morgue until we make a decision. If we decide now, and if we make a phone call now, maybe they can come and pick him up while we're here."

I was in such a daze that I couldn't seem to bring my mind to focus on the necessary details of funeral arrangements. Nevertheless, over the next several days we would have to address the undesirable, yet unavoidable, task of planning a funeral for our son while walking around in a grief-induced stupor. For now, we selected a funeral home and Barb left the room to make the phone call.

I remained in the room with our friends. Our words were few. I was standing by the window, still holding David, alternating my gaze from his small face to the broad city-scape below us, feeling in all my senses a striking contrast between reality and unreality — or what I wanted to be an unreality. I wept several times. They did their best to comfort me, but the greatest comfort came from their mere presence, their willingness to be with us at such a devastating moment, to witness our grief, and to share it.

When Barb returned after making the phone call she said someone from the funeral home would arrive in about a half hour to pick up David. I returned David to her arms. One of our friends called our attention to David's face. We looked down at him and seemed to see the slight suggestion of a smile. We certainly wanted to interpret it that way, even though it could have been the loss of muscle control. Sometime later, Barb related this incident to a friend, who said the smile probably appeared at the moment he met Jesus.

"He's cold, "Barb said, wrapping his blanket a little higher around his chest, as though it would help. Our friends said goodbye to David and left us alone. We sat in the rocking chairs and passed the next thirty minutes or so staring at our son, occasionally breaking the silence to comment about him or to cry. Finally, a nurse entered the room to inform us that the funeral home's transport vehicle had arrived. Barb pressed David closely and kissed him, then placed him in the nurse's arms. She stood there holding him, apparently waiting for us to leave the room. We rose from our chairs. As we approached the door, I turned around, bent down, and kissed David on his forehead. "Goodbye, pal," I whispered.

Barb and I were overwhelmed by the difficulty of that moment, the finality of it. We picked up the empty infant seat that we had brought to the hospital for his comfort. As we held hands and walked out the hospital entrance into the glaring August sunlight, the world seemed even less real. We were lightheaded, bewildered. There was a sense of surprise that everything was still in motion: cars moving down the street, people on the sidewalk, the outdoor sounds of man and nature. Our son had just died. It seemed only right that there should be a pause, a hushed stillness everywhere. But instead, the world around us was going on, as if it had missed the terrible news.

What we were feeling was only the beginning of a sluggish, agonizing process of absorbing our loss and re-emerging into that world that seemed so strange and distant to us right now. Those steps from the hospital to the parking deck were only a fraction of the long journey ahead.

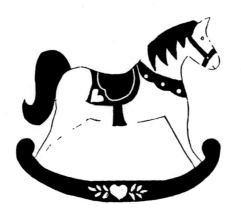

Chapter
Seven

When we arrived home, Barb's parents were there with Steven. Her mother was frantically cleaning the house from top to bottom and catching up on laundry. It was all she could do to occupy her mind. As long as she stayed in motion she could fortify herself against her tremendous grief. Yet, I know that David occupied her every thought.

My own parents, having received the bad news, were by now en route from Buffalo, New York, where they had been spending a few days visiting my two brothers and their families. On the day before they had planned to leave for this trip my mother was debating whether or not to cancel it. She was very concerned about David's sickness. I reassured her that David would be fine in a few days, that there was no reason to cancel the trip. Now they were coming home for their grandson's funeral.

Katie had stayed overnight at a friend's house. As yet, neither she nor Steven knew their brother had died. Barb left to pick her up. I stayed at home, thinking nervously how best to tell the children. I felt sure that Steven, age three, could not fully grasp it. But I could not predict how Katie would understand and react to the loss. My stomach had been tight all morning. But when Barb and Katie returned I could feel it clenching even tighter.

We brought Katie and Steven into the living room to "have a talk". Katie sat on the couch between Barb and me, while Steven stood in front of us. Katie was smiling at the notion of being included in this little "talk," as though she were part of a conspiracy. Then Barb began:

"Katie, do you remember when I explained to you how sick David was, and that he might have to stay in the hospital for a little while?"
Katie nodded, still smiling.
"Well, David won't be coming home, honey. He died this morning."

The smile immediately left Katie's face, replaced by a look of terrible shock. She burst into tears. Barb and I together hugged her and cried with her.

"I'm so sorry we had to tell you this, Katie," I said.

Steven, looking confused and bewildered, joined in our embrace. I cried not only for our loss, but for these two surviving children whom we loved so much, and who had to learn at a young, innocent age the cruelty of life, the reality of death.

Before we had broken the news, I was uncertain of how well Katie would understand the concept of death. Could she conceive and accept the fact that her brother was permanently out of her life — here one day and suddenly gone the next? And Steven, who was obviously too young to have any real notion of death — how could we explain to him in uncomplicated terms what happened to his brother? Their learning process began with that brief, shocking moment, but would continue in the coming days with the calling hours, the funeral, and the burial of their brother's ashes; in the coming months as we grieved painfully over his death; and in the coming years, as we would commemorate him in so many ways. For now, it was important for Barb and me to assure them that David was with God, in heaven, the happiest of all places.

The rest of the day became a blur of activities. More phone calls had to be made to friends and relatives. By mid-afternoon my parents arrived directly from Buffalo at our doorstep. As they entered, they embraced us and shared our tears. We sat down with them and retold the events of the last few days. They praised us for the care we'd given David over the years, and offered their help and support. By late afternoon the news of David's death had spread quickly. There was the intermittent arrival of friends at our door bearing cards and notes, flowers, casseroles, desserts — the traditional expressions of sympathy from those close to us who care, who ached for us, and who knew no better way to show their condolence than to simply be there for us. Their presence and their kind gestures provided comfort for Barb and me. Instead of being alone, we had others to share our grief with, to listen as we told and retold the events of David's sickness and death, and to embrace us as we wept. Their support felt good. I realized then — and even more now — how important it was.

Later that afternoon Barb and I made some decisions. Among them was the decision to have David's body cremated. We also scheduled the calling hours for Thursday evening and the funeral mass for Friday morning. The calling hours would not allow for a final viewing of David, since his body had to be cremated within twenty-four hours after his death or else be embalmed. Yet we wanted at least Katie and Steven, our families, and David's school teachers to have the opportunity to see him one last time. Therefore, we made hasty arrangements for them to gather at the funeral home that evening.

While Barb was upstairs getting ready for the gathering, I was in the kitchen fixing a quick dinner for Katie and Steven. Katie asked me, "Will David live at the funeral home? Can we visit him whenever we want to?"

Her question was both innocent and urgent, demanding both an honest answer and an explanation. I explained to her again that David's soul had already left his body and was living in heaven, that his body was now a lifeless form. I reminded her about a dead bird she and some of the neighborhood kids had found earlier that week and buried in the backyard. Just as we bury animals when they die, because they decay, we have to dispose of human beings when they die, too. I told her we do this in one of two ways: we either bury them in the ground or cremate them — that is, burn their bodies and bury the ashes. I assured her that there is no pain involved in cremation because the body's life is gone. I was sure that the idea of cremation was difficult to understand, and that it seemed strange, perhaps even cruel. But I also knew it was important for her to know what finally happened to her brother, how he was laid to rest. In short, my feelings were ambivalent: on the one hand, I preferred that she didn't know of David's cremation because she probably wouldn't understand; on the other hand, I wanted to be honest and straightforward with her, and not leave the issue unresolved. I did not want to shock or frighten her, but I didn't want her to be confused or deluded about the finality of her brother's death, either. I tried to help her realize that after tonight she would never see him again.

That evening, our families and two of David's teachers gathered at the funeral home. Katie brought with her the get-well gift she had made for David. Barb and I took the children into the viewing room first, in order to have some time alone as a family. Ever since we had left him at the hospital that morning I had been aching for this moment to see him again. There he was at the front of the room, laid upon a sort of cushioned table that was draped with full-length white bunting. Under his head was the Winnie the Pooh pillow he had slept on every night for years. He was dressed in the outfit that had been our favorite, because he looked so boyish, so handsome in it. Death had not diminished that impression, although now his body was cold and had a white, waxy pallor to it. Katie laid her gift beside him. Barb placed a folding chair next to the table, picked David up, and sat with him on her lap. We both kissed him and stroked his hair, trying to encourage Katie and Steven to do the same. But Katie did not want to touch her brother. She seemed somewhat frightened.

"I don't want to burn him," she said.
"What do you mean, Katie?" Barb asked. "You won't burn him if you touch him."

Then it occurred to me what Katie meant: she did not want David to be cremated. Apparently my earlier explanation had not been enough to reassure Katie that cremation was not some painful, unthinkable procedure. But is there really any explanation sufficient enough for a young child who has at least a limited experience of the hurt that results from burns? I told Barb about the conversation Katie and I had earlier, and we reopened the subject with her. We explained that David had left his body and gone to heaven. He no longer needed or wanted his body, and it could no longer feel pain. Although Katie seemed to accept our explanation, she still did not want to touch him. Barb and I wanted badly for her to have some physical contact with her brother, because we felt it would contribute, perhaps in some ritualistic way, to her understanding and acceptance of his death and her ability to express her own farewell to him. But we could not — and would not — pressure her.

Steven, on the other hand, willingly touched and stroked David, but he did not want to hold him. I then took David in my arms and held him. We sat a while longer, talking with the children about David, how special he was, and emphasizing how special they were for having been a loving brother and sister.

Then I returned David to Barb and opened the door to allow the others to come into the room. David's teachers and each member of our families had the opportunity to hold him. There were a lot of tears and embraces. There was also a heartfelt comfort in this gathering of people who had shared David's life, who had loved him, and would now miss him. Together, we were sharing genuinely and intimately the tremendous grief and hurt that had only begun impacting our lives in these early hours after his death. We all spoke freely about his life and death, bolstering each other, partaking of each other's strength.

Toward the end of the evening Steven asked if he could hold David. Barb sat him down on the end of a sofa and laid David across his lap, with his head resting on the sofa's arm. Steven talked to him and gently patted his chest. Finally, Katie, too, expressed a desire to hold her brother. "Are you sure?" Barb asked. Katie nodded. She sat on the sofa, and Barb placed David in her arms. At that moment, Barb and I knew that what we had done for our children, family and friends that evening was the right thing to do. It was good and healthy for all of us. As we watched Steven and Katie holding their brother like they had so many times in his life, our eyes were tearful, but our hearts were full. They were saying goodbye.

Before leaving the funeral home, Barb and I went into the funeral director's office to make arrangements for David's cremation the following day and for calling hours on the following Thursday evening. As we rose from our chairs to leave, Barb opened her purse, pulled something out, and handed it to the director. "Would you please make sure that this goes with David tomorrow?" she asked. "Certainly," he replied, taking it from her. It was the "get well" gift that Katie had made for David.

The following evening, two close friends of ours made an hour-long drive to our home to be with us. Their daughter had been a friend of mine for about five years, until she was tragically and suddenly killed in an automobile accident. They had come to us this evening because they knew — they understood — the terrible pain of our loss, and they wanted to support us. We spent the evening talking with them about our feelings, our grief, our memories. It was a great comfort to talk with them and to explore this strong, common bond of loss. They required no explanations: they had been where we were now. And their love, their concern, their sense of needing to be there for us was a great solace.

The next few days were busy ones, even though they seemed to go by slowly. We had to purchase a cemetery plot for the burial of David's ashes. It was one of those details I really did not want to tend to, because it would only bring me closer to my grief, but it had to be done. Fortunately, a neighbor of ours had a brother who owned several plots in the cemetery where we wanted to bury David, and he kindly offered to sell us one. Going there to look it over was a strange, unreal experience. A salesman drove us through the maze of roads that crisscrossed the cemetery. It was a hot afternoon. I remember wondering, as we passed hundreds of graves, how many of these were the graves of children. How did they die? Did their parents survive the terrible grief? When we arrived at the prospective site, we got out of the car to look at it. It was a beautiful, grassy area of the cemetery, with a cluster of three tall arborvitae trees near the grave and a huge pin oak close by. We both liked the idea — or perhaps the metaphor — of David's final resting place being under the shade and protection of tall trees. Within walking distance was a duck pond fed by a stream. We had wanted David to be buried close to Barb's and my future grave sites. So we decided to purchase a plot for two — for Barb and me — and David's ashes would be buried at the head of the plot, directly below the marker.

The next day, we went to our church to plan a liturgy for David's memorial mass. A liturgist helped us sort through the many prayers and scriptural readings that would be appropriate, and Barb and I made final selections. A musician also gave us a sizeable catalog of songs and hymns to choose from. In addition, we composed two prayers of our own to be read at the mass. When we finished, we felt good about the liturgy we had designed. It seemed to reflect so much of David's innocence, his life, his difficult journey in this world, as well as celebrating his new life with God. This mass was important to us because it would be the last farewell to David from his relatives and friends. It would be a celebration of his life with us. It would be our message to him and to God. And it would be God's message to all of us.

That evening, Barb asked me how far I had progressed in the construction of a rocking horse I had begun building for David a couple of months earlier. During the past year we had put a lot of work into remodeling David's bedroom, and Barb had begun decorating it in a rocking horse theme. That's when I had decided to build a large classical-styled rocking horse. I knew that David would never be able to ride it, but it would be a wonderful decoration for his bedroom.

Now, Barb wondered if I could at least finish the construction of it by Thursday evening, so we could display it, along with many of our favorite pictures and mementos of David, at the calling hours. So I spent the next two days patiently cutting and shaping the remaining pieces, assembling legs to torso, putting the eyes into the sockets, mounting the horse to its rockers, and sanding, sanding, sanding. As I worked, I thought about David. I thought about the excitement with which Barb and I had undertaken the remodeling of his bedroom in a desire to make it special for him.

I remembered the stacks of wallpaper sample books that Barb had brought home and flipped through, over and over, to find the perfect print and color. I remembered the day we completed the stripping and staining of the woodwork. I remembered the frustration of installing carpet for the first time. I remembered Barb's enthusiasm in shopping for all of the special decorations she had chosen for the room. The original enthusiasm I had for this rocking horse project was gone. After all, it was to be my personal gift to David, and now he was gone. In place of that enthusiasm, however, was a strong desire to commemorate him in my craftsmanship. I dedicated my labor to him, as though competing with the quality of every previous project I had ever undertaken. The finished product was beautiful. I was proud of what my hands had done in the name of our son. To this day the rocking horse remains in the bedroom where he slept, a kind of monument to his memory.

On Thursday we went to the funeral home early. We placed the rocking horse at the front of the receiving area. Also at front were a beautiful portrait of David as an infant that my sister had rendered in charcoal, and a poem I had written three years earlier. A friend of ours had generously reproduced the poem in calligraphy and framed it for us on only a day's notice. Around the room, on tables and furniture, we displayed other pictures, albums and mementos of David.

All week long we had, in a way, gravitated toward this evening. It would be the opportunity for us to be comforted by so many people who knew us and who knew David. Their presence would be a tribute to our son.

If we were moved by the expressions of sympathy that had come to our door in the last five days, we were overwhelmed by this huge gathering of friends and relatives who had come to express their respect for David and their sympathy for us. Barb and I stood at the front of the room with Katie and Steven. But as more and more people arrived, we separated and began making the rounds, so that we would be able to greet everyone. The sight of so many people warmed our hearts. Even more warming was the presence of those we least expected to see, people with whom we'd had little or no contact over the years. The kind words that were spoken that night, the gestures, the embraces were so important and gratifying to us. Many who were there told us their personal stories or memories of David. They soothed the terrible aching within us, if only for a while, and reminded us of how many lives our little son — who never spoke or communicated — had touched.

The next day, Friday, was David's memorial mass. I woke up that morning feeling an additional sadness, knowing that this day would be the final goodbye to our son. Afterwards, everyone would go home. There would be no more funeral or calling hours, no spontaneous visitors at the door bearing gifts or expressions of sympathy, no one to weep with us. The sympathy cards and notes would slow to a trickle, then one day stop. And we would be left with the enormous task of trying to put our lives back on track, to reintegrate ourselves back into the everyday world. At this point in time, the task seemed impossible.

The funeral mass was celebrated by a priest who is a good friend of ours. He went out of his way, both in the mass and in his sermon, to make this a profound and personal celebration of David's life. His words were well-chosen, sympathetic and poignant. He spoke of the relevance of David's life to the message God has for all of us. He reminded us that we, as human beings, are all "handicapped", in some sense of the word, by our own selfishness, pettiness or cruelty toward one another. He offered the assurance that David's life had a profound purpose that somehow glorified God. And, finally, he praised our family — each of us in a personal way, then all of us together — for the love we shared and the care we had given to David.

Before the final blessing and closing of the mass Barb stood up in the front of the church and read a poem I had written about David two years earlier. It was something special she wanted to do, knowing I was unable to do it. She had asked my older brother to stand beside her, ready to take over in case she would have

trouble finishing the reading. As she began to read, Steven —
before I could stop him — left our pew, walked to the front of the
church, and stood beside his mother, facing the congregation.
Perhaps his innocent gesture gave Barb strength. She not only read
the entire poem, but rendered it so beautifully that many in the
church were in tears, including me.

Following the mass we all gathered in the church hall for a
meal. Barb and I had chosen not to bury David's ashes on the
same day as the funeral. That would be another day, with a private
ceremony to include just the four of us. In the meantime, the urn
that contained his remains would be held at the funeral home.

The funeral plans had been fulfilled, and the many who had
come to pay their respects went home. In the days following there
was a profound nothingness, a self-conscious silence. Perhaps our
grief was already progressing from its incipient trauma stage to
one of passive incredulity.

To contemplate life without David was unimaginable. The
absence of our son seemed to glare back at us everywhere we
looked. There were so many visible reminders — his clothes, his
toys, his bedroom, his special feeding tray, jars of strained food in
the cupboard. All of these became emblems of our separation from
David and sometimes intensified our sense of loss. Especially
painful were the photographs of him that we had displayed in
several rooms of the house. Each picture seemed to capture his
wide-eyed innocence in a way that sometimes moved me to tears.
Would I ever be able to "let go" of him? It seemed not. And as I
thought about the life that lay ahead of me, it was with feelings of
emptiness, even fear.

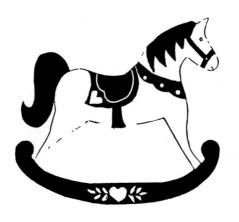

Chapter
Eight

We seemed to be walking in a fog. David was our first thought upon waking, our last before falling asleep, and almost our only thought during the day. It was as though our minds had become a kind of chamber, resonating with all the emotions we connected to our son. His death was still an incredible shock that we couldn't quite fully absorb. There was now an emptiness in our home and in our lives that could not be bridged or filled. It was there forever. Barb and I often discussed our grieving thoughts and cried together. The enormity of this pain and its all-encompassing quality made our spirits heavy. There were moments when I felt compelled to draw in a deep breath — as if I were suffocating — and then let it out in a sigh. And yet, in an odd way, the grieving felt good. It kept us focused on David. It was now the only way we had of expressing our love for him. Beside the memories, it was all we had left of him. At the time, the idea of relinquishing that grief seemed the moral equivalent of relinquishing everything about David: life, memories, legacy — everything! Therefore, the grief was something to hold on to, a kind of life raft amidst the wreckage. However, it was also an impediment to carrying on with our daily lives in a meaningful fashion.

Though Barb and I grieved together, we also grieved separately. At times, this created an accumulation of unspoken stress and frustration in our relationship that was difficult to deal with openly and honestly. There were certain feelings and emotions we expressed to each other, but, once expressed, they became redundant. Each of us knew the other's pain, but each of us was being consumed by our own unbearable pain. There were differences in the patterns and themes of our grief, as well as in the personal expression they nurtured. After all, there were thoughts, memories and emotions that were intrinsically our own. One of mine was the frequent mental flashbacks of David's last moments. The witnessing of my son's death left a powerful memory that could not be shaken. And with its playback came the incredulity, the fear, the helplessness, the tremendous sadness that had washed over me during the actual event. This memory was my own; no one else shared it. It often left me with feelings of loneliness and despair. Sometimes it led to morbid thoughts and fantasies of losing another of our children. After all, David's death taught us an agonizing lesson: that our lives are fragile and death is random. How could I ever survive the loss of another child?

One of the feelings that Barb struggled with for a long time afterward was a sense of guilt for not having been present when David died. She had been told that David would probably linger for several hours. She called me to his bedside so that we could both be there for him and share what little time was left together. But by the time she returned to the room David had expired, long before the doctor predicted. In Barb's own mind, her absence was tantamount to neglect. It was unforgivable. She was his mother. She knew he was dying. She should have been there to help him, to comfort him, to simply be with him. She felt she had let him down at perhaps the most important moment of his life: his death. Nothing I said could assuage her guilt and remorse. This was an emotional issue that she had to work through on her own. All I could do was offer support and reassurance.

Katie and Steven dealt with their grief far differently than Barb and I. For one thing, they were too young to fully comprehend the mystery of death. Nevertheless, Barb and I were deeply moved by their innocent observations, their expression of feelings, their questions ("When can we visit David again?" "What will he do in heaven?"). Steven never did cry over David's death. Katie did not cry beyond the moment we broke the news to her. Yet Barb and I knew they were working through their own grief, trying to make sense of their brother's absence. I think that their emotions sometimes hinged on ours. They were saddened by the sight of Barb or me crying, or by sensing our sorrow and depression. At times it was difficult to tend to their emotional needs because we were so preoccupied with our own deep pain. For this reason, we felt obligated to explain to them how much we were hurting, and that we still loved them, even if we sometimes failed to show it. We encouraged them to talk about David's death whenever they raised the issue. We tried to draw out their true feelings and make them feel comfortable with those emotions. But most of all, we continually tried to instill in them a sense that they were special for having shared as brother and sister the life and love of their disabled brother.

In general, Katie and Steven bounced back into their daily lives in a relatively short time. Sometimes, this made me feel almost resentful. How could they forget their brother's death so soon? But, at the same time, I realized that children have an amazing resiliency to such shock and pain. Sorrow does not linger as long with them, nor penetrate every aspect of their lives. They are insulated from the cruelties of life by their own innocence, their natural naivete -- and that is as it should be.

In the wake of David's death, Katie and Steven became all the more precious to us. Sometimes I would look at them and feel a surge of emotion that prompted me to hug or kiss them, or show some sign of affection. For a long while Barb and I became cautious and protective of them, fearing they could be injured — or worse — at play or other activities. Whenever they did get hurt or become sick, it alarmed us more sharply than before. Not that we wanted to spoil them or protect them to the point of isolation, but we both had in our heads this fear — however rational or irrational — that we could lose another child. And inside that fear was another, more subliminal one: the dread that a second loss would absolutely destroy us. It was a fear that we readily admitted and discussed with each other, but one that took a long time to overcome.

A week after David's death I returned to work. It was really the last place I wanted to be. The job, like so many other things, now seemed so trivial and unimportant. But if I had taken more time off, I would only have wallowed in pain at home. Returning to work was the right thing for me to do — I somehow knew that, but I didn't want to believe it.

I felt strange being back on the job. It was difficult to function mentally, to organize and orchestrate the day's activities. David was on my mind constantly. My body seemed to be on "automatic pilot". If I stopped thinking of him for several minutes, I would

119

feel amazed and guilty for such lapses when he returned to my thoughts. Sometimes the emotions I was experiencing were so intense, it was as if I could physically feel them welling inside me. Only a few of my co-workers made mention of my son's death. On the other hand, they acted sympathetically in an awkward sort of way. But all I looked forward to was leaving at the end of the day, returning home, and reading the sympathy cards that had arrived in the day's mail.

After a couple of weeks I was beginning to become accustomed to work again. David still dominated my thoughts, but with a less painful intensity that allowed me to feel more comfortable, more in tune with my work, more focused. I recognized at this point that my job and its daily routine were therapeutic, helping me toward a healing process.

For Barb, my return to work brought more loneliness and emotional strain. With Katie back in school now, Barb and Steven were the only ones at home during the day. Despite his presence, she felt alone and isolated in the house which held so many tangible and intangible memories of David. When I came home from work one day several months after David's death, she informed me that she had gone to a psychologist that afternoon for grief counseling.

"Why, Barb?" I asked. "Is it that bad?"

Apparently I had not been aware of her intensely private struggle, how deeply she was hurting, and how much guilt she had worked up inside.

"Yes," she replied, "it's that bad. I have David on my mind all day long. The regret I feel for not having been with him when he died overwhelms me sometimes. I'm here with him in this house every day. I vacuum and dust his bedroom. I see and I touch things that were his, or were part of his life. The memories, the photographs, the routines that no longer have to be followed — it all makes me ache inside. I feel like I've lost every emotion except my grief. I know you're still hurting, but at least you get out of the house every day and have a job to occupy your mind. I don't have that, so sometimes it seems there's just no escape from my grief. I felt I had to talk to a professional just to see if she could help me. But I'm not going back. I think it was a waste of time."

Barb did not go back for further grief counseling. But she began to respond to the support of a few close friends. One in particular was a friend who had helped us out years before by babysitting David when we had difficulty finding someone willing to babysit a child with his problems. Several times after the diagnosis of David's brain damage, Barb and I had poured our hearts out to her. She was a wonderful listener, warm and genuine, and she was very supportive. David's death was very jarring to her, too. She had come to visit him at the hospital that morning, but arrived too late. After the funeral, she began calling Barb once or more a week to see how she was doing and to lend support. Barb would talk to her about David's death, her own grief, the changes that tragedy had wrought in our lives, sometimes repeating the same conversation time after time. But this friend listened patiently and with great sympathy, offering herself as a sounding board, a shoulder to cry upon. Her friendship and her skills as a good listener and responder became enormously valuable to Barb, and helped her in the healing process.

Part of our mutual healing process involved venturing out beyond the walls of our own home as a family. There was an ambivalence in this that is hard to explain. On the one hand, we wanted to get out and be able to move about among family and friends. But sometimes in the act of doing so, we ended up wishing we had stayed at home — our "grief shelter". Being away from home and out in public sometimes made us feel awkward, as if we were groping somewhere between darkness and light, between the re-entry process and the desire to remain somewhat isolated, keeping our grief alive. Always there was the self-consciousness of being incomplete now as a family — someone was missing. Of course, these feelings were strongest for

Barb and me. Katie and Steven, although they sometimes commented on his absence ("Too bad David can't be with us."), were happy to get out of the house, to go places and do things.

Our first real outing after David's death was a Labor Day family picnic at my sister's home. On her porch was a television set. We were watching the Jerry Lewis Muscular Dystrophy Telethon on and off. At one point, a guest on the show — an older gentleman who had muscular dystrophy — gave an emotional appeal for support. He talked about the personal history of his debilitating disease and about his impending death by it. All eyes were on the T.V. I glanced over at Barb and I could see she was on the verge of tears. We got up from our chairs and walked around the side of the house, where we both broke down and cried. It was one of many such incidents following David's death, especially during that first year. We were learning that healing is an ongoing experience in which the pain may seem to diminish, then suddenly spike again. The loss of a child is a sorrow beyond all comprehension. That sorrow became the essence, indeed the matrix, of our existence. It had an insidious quality that overwhelmed reason and meaning. Yet it had the ability to internalize and interpret experiences and events of everyday life and color them with sadness. The spontaneity of tears and emotions was something we seemed to have little control over. Sometimes triggered by a memory, sometimes by something someone said, or sometimes merely by a good book, a movie or beautiful music, the tears came at unpredictable moments. Our hearts were so vulnerable that any tangible or intangible reminder of our son and of our loss struck a tremendously sensitive nerve.

In social situations we were often uncertain of whether we could feel free to talk about David. We wanted to — sometimes needed to — talk about his death and our grief and the difficulties of carrying on, or to share some memory of him. But it became obvious that, in some company, the topic made people uncomfortable. They did not know how to speak or react, how to engage us. Over time we learned to evaluate social situations before bringing up the subject of David, understanding that we shouldn't think less of others because of their awkwardness or uneasiness. Nor should we mistake their avoidance of the subject as coldness or apathy. Most were sympathetic people who simply found it difficult to express themselves regarding our loss.

Occasionally we would meet up with someone who had not heard the news of David's death. We would retell the details of his final days as if it all had to be retold, not only for the listener's sake, but for our own sakes as well. It rekindled those emotions inside of us, which were perhaps beginning to settle and soften, by confronting us with a rush of memories. On several occasions, friends and family members discovered old photographs of David, which they would give to us either in originals or copies. Any new or unseen or forgotten pictures of our son would stir our very souls with a mixture of enjoyment and pain. Such pictures were surprises and treasures. Some would bring tears, some a chuckle or a memory close to our hearts. Those who gave them could not have imagined what wonderful gifts they had given, nor the depth of our gratitude upon seeing them for the first time.

The time beyond our son's death moved slowly and achingly, each day beginning with the conscious tabulation of time between his death and the present, and ending with the growing awareness, yet disbelief, that we will never experience his physical being again. The onset of the fall and winter seasons seemed the perfect landscape for our emotions: the trees empty of their leaves, the shortening days, the cold, the gray and white colors of the barren winter. It was as though our souls had been externalized.

The loss of David also meant the loss of those daily routines and responsibilities involved in his care: feeding, medicating, diapering, changing clothes, getting him on and off the school bus. Such activities organized and divided the day into a set schedule. Now our days were free of such duties. But we found no relief in that fact. Instead, we would have given anything to be performing those tasks for him. I missed the companionship we shared when I fed him his dinner each evening. At 5:00 p.m. I sometimes felt compelled to plug in his warming tray and fill it with food, though

I never did. And how I missed the feel of his scrawny, naked body against mine under the warm spray of the shower, or his groan of recognition when I would enter his bedroom and say, "Good morning, buddy."

On a deeper level, all of those mundane daily routines had given me a sense of personal worth. I had embraced the conviction that loving and caring for this special child was the best thing I had done with my life. It represented the goodness in me that no one could challenge. But now, with David gone, I had lost that sense of purpose and self-esteem. I could no longer be that person I was. The notion that when you lose a child, you lose a part of yourself is quite true. That almost seamless bond between identity and purpose is suddenly and cruelly severed. I began to question who I am, why I am here, and whether I could find happiness in redefining myself or reinventing a role for myself.

Early one morning several months after David's death, I was standing in front of the bathroom mirror shaving with my electric razor and thinking of him. For some reason my focus shifted from the reflection of my face to that of my eyes staring back at me. I slowly moved the razor away from my face, switched it off, and stared silently into the mirror. The person I was staring at seemed distant, the face of a stranger, yet vaguely familiar. As I studied the eyes, the slight lines of the face, the expression of the mouth, I thought I could see an indwelling pain. It seemed a visage of sorrow from which all other features faded. I felt sorry for this person. I wanted to comfort him. But, after all, that person was me, a lesser self than I had ever been. I switched my razor back on and finished shaving. In this brief encounter I was examining my outward appearance and interpreting its underlying expression. I was seeing my new self -- the bereaved father -- as a stranger, as someone apart, someone I did not know. And there was a kind of grief in that, too. This strangeness, this effort to grasp the unfamiliar, to comprehend, to make sense of my life and the events that impinged upon it was one of the themes of my grief that cropped up again and again.

During his lifetime I had written poems about David. Now I found myself once again putting pen to paper. The act of writing became a kind of therapy for me. In it I found comfort and expression. It allowed me to externalize my emotions and explore their deeper meaning. And in my writing I could pay tribute to my son and give testament to who and what he was in my life, an idea that seemed more important to me now than ever before.

My brother-in-law, who had lost his father a couple of years earlier, told me that the first year between David's death and the anniversary of his death would be the most difficult. He was right. After the funeral, after the burial, after the last sympathy card, we found ourselves alone, trying to deal with our grief in the absence of all that collective support. There is truly nothing to compare this to. The breadth and complexity of our emotions was bewildering even to us Without David, life was both different and difficult. The emptiness inside us was so pervasive that it robbed us of motivation. Everyday routines sometimes required enormous effort. We couldn't seem to care about so many of the things to which we had previously attached a greater or lesser importance. Household chores, repairs, woodworking projects, things that once filled our days and kept our lives busy were now either abandoned or undertaken half-heartedly. We now felt a disinclination toward such things. No endeavor seemed worth the effort.

Even months after his death we were still feeling a sense of shock and numbness. Inasmuch as we began carrying on with our daily lives, we seemed detached from the world. Memories of David, both bitter and sweet, seemed to resonate in our minds constantly. Like the winter season, our grief was settling in, deepening. It was hard to feel happy, or even contented. Nor did we feel excitement or find anything worthy of looking forward to. Instead, we were immersed in a mood of melancholy and contemplation. Barb and I both began reading books on death and the grieving process, if only to reassure ourselves that we were not going crazy. We discovered that all of these feelings, moods and emotions we were experiencing were quite normal for bereaved parents. We were simply grappling with the most wrenching of all realities — the death of our child. For years we had known that David would not have a long life. But that knowledge did not seem to change our perspective on his death. It was still shocking and unreal. We yearned for him. We wanted him back. I have heard it said that the loss of a child is the worst tragedy that life can hand to us, and Barb and I found that to be so. Nothing can shock us more, nothing can hurt us more, nothing can change our lives more profoundly and irreversibly. And amid the depression and soul-searching was the formidable, painful, persistent question: "Why?" I thought of the many sicknesses that David had survived in his short life. Why did this one have to be the final one? There are no answers. Or perhaps the questions are the answers — the revelation that life is a mystery that we cannot fully know or understand or even grasp.

In the midst of our inertia and apathy we were also reflecting on our own lives. I often wondered what was the purpose of David's short, difficult life. I questioned my faith. I questioned God — or whether there truly was a God. If so, was he involved in our lives? Did his hand move events on this earth, or simply set it into a spinning motion like a top, only to abandon it? Did God care about us? If so, how could he justify David's life and death and all the resulting heartbreak they wrought in our lives? Did he bring David into the world to inspire a special love in us, only to take him away from us? And if, in fact, there is no God, then our lives are merely biological accidents or events. I often reflected on my own mortality, as well as that of my wife and children. Any one of us could be gone without a moment's notice, powerless in the face of death. We live and we die — all to what purpose? At the deepest of my depression I was sometimes convinced that life was devoid of meaning. And this conclusion, in itself, brought on another kind of grief that only added to my sense of darkness and emptiness. It was only after giving up the questioning that the answers slowly began to come in the years ahead, through events that seemed to reveal a genuine purpose in David's life and in our family.

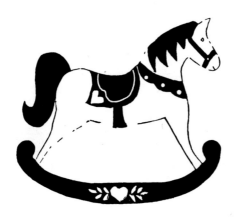

Chapter
Nine

128

The day that David died became a reference point in time. In the early weeks and months, we mentally marked off another week for each Sunday that passed, noting the precise moment he died. The connections between the day of his death and the past or present sometimes manifested themselves in the most trivial ways. For example, I would open the cupboard or the freezer and recall that a particular food item was purchased before he died. Or one autumn day, while installing a storm window in David's bedroom, I noted that the last time I performed this seasonal ritual my son was alive. Or sometimes just being at a certain place would cause me to remember that the last time I'd been there was before that day of that month of that year of his death. There's no making sense of how pervasively the mind tracks such little, inconsequential things. Perhaps the reason time became divided into "before his death" and "after his death" stemmed from the perception of distance between who I had been and who I was now. This figurative revisitation of situations and places confronted me with my old self — the happy father who had a son named David — standing on the other side of an enormous gulf. It was like a subliminal awareness of a part of my past I could no longer possess or even reach, and it sometimes made me ache. I don't know whether to describe that ache as a feeling or as simply the loss of feeling. But I was unable to imagine life becoming happy and fulfilling again. I wanted to go back to the past.

That day, that month, that year also became the landmark to which I related the placing of many other events, both large and small, into the span of time. My mind subconsciously catalogued many things relative to time before or after his death. To this day I still recall events as having occurred within that frame of reference.

Among the events that brought our grief sharply into focus were the annual holidays. We had always spent them together with one or both of our families, and David had always been included in those holiday gatherings. Because I come from a family of ten, those gatherings tended to be large. For that reason, David enjoyed a variety of laps and shoulders, as everyone took turns holding him. Their acceptance of David was wonderful, and it gave us a good feeling. But now, we were no longer bringing David to holiday parties. Instead, we were bringing our own emptiness, our self-conscious feelings of incompleteness. For Barb and I, those special days of the year took on a different mood, one of longing, as we remembered how they had been celebrated in years past with David in our midst. We approached each holiday not with the usual anticipation of festivities, but rather with the purpose of getting through it, and doing so without openly displaying our grief in ways that would make others uncomfortable. For us, the only important aspect of each holiday was how to commemorate David on that day.

On the first Thanksgiving after his death, we visited his grave and laid flowers there. The bronze grave marker we had ordered was now in place and we saw it for the first time. David's name and dates stood out in bold relief, flanked on either side by Barb's and mine. It was an official, yet inadequate, monument to our son. Nothing about who he was, what he endured in his short life, or how much he meant to those who loved him. Strange, too, for Barb and I to stare at our own names, along with our dates of birth, followed by that blank space waiting to be filled in. We held hands and stared quietly for a while, stifling our tears. Then we all got back into the car and drove to Barb's parents for Thanksgiving dinner.

As the Christmas holidays approached, Katie and Steven exhibited all the anticipation and excitement of children their age. It was an enthusiasm that Barb and I could not seem to enter into and share with them. But we didn't want to dampen their spirits or ruin what, for them, was the happiest, most long-awaited day of the entire year. So we summoned our efforts to make this holiday a happy one for our children and a meaningful one for all of us. We bought gifts. Barb purchased the first of many rocking horse ornaments we would hang on our Christmas tree to commemorate David. She found a miniature Christmas tree, which we decorated and placed on his grave. But when the time came to put up our own Christmas tree, Barb expressed a lack of enthusiasm about doing so. "Why don't we forget the tree this year," she said. "I'm just not in the mood for it." I knew exactly what she meant, because I felt the same way. But then an idea struck. "Why don't we put the tree in David's bedroom this year?" I said. She looked at me as though I were crazy. A few days later, I arrived home from work and found that she had rearranged the furniture in his room to clear a space for the tree.

And so, on that first Christmas morning without him, we gathered in David's bedroom not only to celebrate, but to remember someone who was an important part of Christmases gone by. Before opening gifts, Barb and I read aloud a card which all of us had signed, and in which I had written a short letter to David. Then Barb passed to me a small wrapped package to open. Inside the wrapping was the miniature rocking horse ornament she had bought. I stood up and hung it proudly from a branch of the tree. Although this Christmas and the ones to come could never be the same, we had found some means of coping, of getting beyond that proverbial "lump in the throat" by translating our sorrow into a shared and meaningful expression.

After what seemed a long time beyond Christmas came David's birthday, February 16th, 1988. Again, we felt the need to acknowledge this day in some special way. But, at the same time, we were painfully aware of the irony of celebrating the birthday of a child who is no longer with us. As the date approached, my thoughts turned to that day nine years ago, when he was born. It was such a happy day, a new beginning for us. Indeed, a new beginning that would take a bitter twist.

I awoke early on the morning of what would have been David's ninth birthday. I pulled from the bookshelf the two large photo albums we had filled with photos of him. With those and a cup of coffee I sat down alone in his bedroom and flipped through page after page of those moments, sometimes sobbing, sometimes smiling. How important these pictures, these still-life fragments of his existence had become! They were memories, pieces of human time tenderly collated and preserved. There were photographs of him in the intensive care unit taken days after his birth, his homecoming, his first bath, his baptism, his first haircut, birthdays, favorite outfits, therapy sessions, school activities and field trips. There were pictures of him sitting on Santa's lap; of Barb stroking his hand across the back of a baby goat at the petting zoo; of me floating him in the water of a warm pool; and of him with his brother and sister, friends, relatives and teachers. Many of the pictures drew my memory back to the event, the situation, the day they were taken, sometimes recalling the mood or emotion. Those photographs, and the proximity of the memories they inspired, made his absence seem all the more unbelievable.

Later that day we visited his grave and placed flowers there. Katie, all on her own, had made a card to accompany the flowers. We joined hands and sang "Happy Birthday" to David. As we turned to walk back to the car, Katie said, "Wait! Can I read my card?" "Certainly," Barb told her. The words she read aloud were short, simple, and yet, profound for such a young child:

"Dear Jesus, help us understand why David died and why we all have to die."

Barb and I, struck by the poignancy of her words, could only compliment her on writing such a wonderful card. She smiled proudly.

That evening, we had a birthday dinner in David's honor, complete with cake and candles. Each of us signed our name to a card, which we displayed on the refrigerator door.

In many similar ways we observed other holidays and special events throughout that first year. Often our mourning was — and still is — expressed as the need to commemorate David in small ways. The year following his death we made many trips to the cemetery — sometimes as a family, sometimes the two of us, or sometimes one of us alone. His grave was one place where I could still feel his presence in a comforting kind of way, as though I could commune with him.

Some days I would go out for early morning walks to spend time thinking about him and talking to him mentally. There were also mornings when I would go into his bedroom while everyone was still asleep and sit in the rocking chair. On one such occasion, I tried to imagine him there in his crib, waking up. I bent over the rail and pretended to lift him and hold him against my chest, my arms wrapping him as if they remembered their exact position, my shoulder lifting slightly as though it were supporting his head at rest there. And with focused intensity I pretended to carry him out of the bedroom and down the hallway, as I had done so often. For only a few brief seconds, it felt like I had my son back again. The moment was unreal but, at the same time, deliberate and willful. It was just one of those rare, unexplainable occasions when I felt compelled to act out or ritualize my longing in a private and personal expression.

The weeks and months of that first year seemed to pass slowly, but we were, nevertheless, cognizant of their passing. They opened ever wider the gulf between the present and the day of our son's death. There was a feeling of regret in this — that we were moving farther in time from that tragic day. Even in the dark and seemingly timeless labyrinth of emotions that contained us there had been an odd kind of comfort in feeling the nearness of our tragedy. It was important to us. We clung to it because it amplified all of the emotional ties we still had to David. It connected us in a way that nothing else could anymore. By now we had accepted his death. We had experienced the realness of his lifeless body, his funeral, his burial, his name in the obituary, his daily absence from our lives. We had experienced the isolation, the emotional exhaustion, the near-desperation that accompanies such acceptance. But we discovered that beyond the phase of resignation and acceptance lies a more immense task: that of letting go. Finding the ability to resolve our grief, to leave David in the past, and to give structure to our strange, new lives was the most demanding work of our hearts and minds.

Perhaps that was part of the reason why, in June, 1988, Barb and I made an appointment with David's doctor. We wanted to talk with him about David's final days, not to re-live them, but to order up the events of his sickness, to understand their cause-and-effect progression, and to finally lay them to rest. The doctor began by, once again, expressing his sympathy for our loss and commending us for the care and devotion we had given David throughout his lifetime. He asked us how we were coping. We talked for a little while about our grief and about the adjustments David's death had wrought in our lives. He commented that David's life was surely prolonged by our love. It was strange to hear a doctor speak in such genuine, human, non-medical terms, but it was also comforting. This was the person who had helped us steer David through so many crises with his knowledge of medical science.

Attesting to that fact was the bulging file folder he held on his lap, with the name"Greenwald, David" printed on the tab and the word "Deceased" written across the front cover. Everything in that folder was now nothing but history—merely academic. The battle for David's life had finally been lost, and nothing in those medical records could describe that loss in its sharpest and most personal terms.

After answering questions about David's last days he handed the file over to us. We took it home and read through the it. There were many letters written between David's doctors. This one from his first neurologist caught my eye and I read it with interest.

Dear Dr. ____

David Greenwald, age 18 months, son of Robert and Barbara Greenwald, was seen for follow up on October 2, 1980 because of his microcephaly, seizures and marked developmental retardation.

This youngster continues to struggle along and has made rather little developmental progress. His seizures continue in spite of the use of Phenobarbital, 10 mg, and Dilantin, 24 mg. Both of these medications are being administered in therapeutic dosage and the most recent serum levels were within the therapeutic range.

On examination David remains a markedly micro-cephalic, spastic and retarded infant. I noted several brief seizures during the time he was in the office...

In summary, I think David remains a very badly damaged youngster and his prognosis for the future remains bleak...

Of all the letters in the folder this one struck me the most because it was so shocking, yet so clinically honest and accurate. The folder was also packed with medical correspondence and lab reports and discharge summaries describing heart defects, seizures, viral infections, pneumonia, congestive heart failure, micro-cephaly, brain damage and cerebral palsy—in short, the whole spectrum of maladies and episodes that plagued his short life, some of which I had forgotten. And there on the last line of the last page of the last discharge report, dated 8-16-87, appeared this summation: "...the patient was pronounced dead at 10:15 a.m."

What more could be said?

The remaining months of that summer seemed to pass more quickly. We found ourselves counting down the weeks and days leading up to the one-year anniversary of David's death. It seemed incredible that an entire year had passed. Considering all the emotional turbulence we had been through in that span of time, I found myself somewhat in awe that I had made it through. A year ago I couldn't have been sure how long or how well I would bear up under the sorrow that life had placed on our shoulders. In fact, I could not—and did not want to —imagine the future at all. But now it was here and with it came some feelings of regret. That stretch of time between David's death and the anniversary of his death was like a cocoon for us. We endured all of those special "first" occasions and events without him. We spent the year remembering him, grieving for him, and creatively commemorating him in our own ways. Our loss had a sense of immediacy about it. But time had come full circle, and moving beyond that first year represented, for us, a kind of breaking out of that cocoon. We could no longer mark time in the same way now, or anticipate a first holiday without him. It had already been done. We expected that beyond this first year there would be a lessening of the heartache, a leaving behind of much of the emotional baggage that grief had encumbered us with. But would we also be leaving behind our son? So much of our love for David and our memories of him had been manifested in our grief. As that grief diminished, would the love, the memories, the importance of David in our lives diminish in a proportionate manner? Such questions and uncertainties gave us an ambivalent outlook toward this one-year anniversary. If this day was to mark a kind of new beginning, a healing, a going forward at the price of forgetting or depreciating our son, then it seemed unworthy of our observance. David was very important to us. But what we would soon realize is that these questions and uncertainties we were experiencing were the beginning of a resolution of our grief. They represented our search for a balance between past and present and at least a desire to feel hopeful about the future.

On the anniversary day, August 16, we went to the cemetery to visit David's grave and to lay flowers on it. We had also invited our families and some close friends to join us. We hadn't planned any kind of ceremony, but we simply wanted their presence, their support, their remembrance. Most of them had never been to the cemetery (David's burial had been a private ceremony.) We wanted everyone to see his final resting place.

We emerged from our cars into the bright morning sun, gathering around the grave and talking to one another. Then Barb and I moved to the front of the marker and stood silently staring down at it, each absorbed in our own thoughts. The conversation around us began to quiet down. As I stared, I was thinking about that day one year ago as if it were yesterday. I recalled Barb's urgent phone call from the hospital. I remembered David's face, and the slowing of his heartbeat under my hand. And I remembered looking out the window of his hospital room at the buildings and the streets below as I held his lifeless body in my arms. Barb and I suddenly joined hands, then broke into sobs, then embraced. We spoke no words to each other. We didn't have to.

We both knew what a monumental moment this was for each of us, what it had taken for us to come this far, having journeyed through the unfathomable heartbreak, desolation, loneliness and longing known only by those who have lost a child. After we dried our eyes, everyone formed a circle around the grave and, with hands joined, recited a prayer.

That afternoon the four of us went swimming at a nearby lake, along with two of David's former teachers. We passed the afternoon enjoying the water and the conversation, much of it centering on memories of our son. We chose that activity because we didn't want this to be an emotionally gloomy day. We wanted it to be a happy one, spent together with our children. In the passing of that day, Barb and I both recognized its importance and sensed in it a new beginning. There was a feeling of relief from the anticipation that had accompanied the approach of the anniversary. Indeed, we somehow knew that the days beyond this would become easier, happier, more filled with the wholeness of living.

As we began the second year after David's death, I could consciously feel the burden of grief lighten. He was still in my thoughts every single day, but no longer dominated them. The sorrow no longer colored my mood. For both of us, the tearful remembrances became fewer and farther between. We were able to dwell more on the fond and happy memories of David's life and less on the sad ones. Our lives seemed to be opening up, renewing themselves. We began going places and doing things more often as a family, some of which we could not have done—or would have been difficult to do—with David. The emotions of laughter and joy began to come more easily. If we were learning to leave David behind, we were not forgetting him. Instead, we were discovering that his life and death had made us emotionally richer. To this day our family commemorations of David often include some verbal or ritualistic remembrance of him, because the idea of keeping his memory alive has become a conviction we embrace with tenderness. During holidays and special times of the year we display pieces of school artwork that David had brought home for

Halloween, Thanksgiving, Christmas, Easter, Valentine's Day, Saint Patrick's Day, Mothers' Day, Fathers' Day or personal occasions. Each Christmas, we purchase a new rocking horse ornament for the tree as a remembrance of him. Some of his possessions we still keep on display as mementos. Following mealtime prayers, we always say, "Hi, David", before we begin eating. Although each holiday observance or celebration has a corresponding somberness, we find each remembrance to be gratifying in its own way, each contributing to our awareness and understanding of the goodness that David has brought into our lives.

It is not as though we have enshrined David. The expressions of remembrance I mentioned above have been part of the ongoing process of mourning, healing and recovery. Those practices that we still hang onto today provide us with a frame of reference, a meaningful connection to someone who was—and still is—a part of our lives. These and other commemorative acts have given us a sense of acceptance toward David's death. They allow us to let go of him and yet hold onto the memories of him and the gifts he has given us. Those will always be a part of us: wherever we go, we take them with us.

Shortly after his death, Barb and I had discussed the possibility of taking in a foster child with disabilities. We felt that David had given us a special experience, a special compassion, and special abilities that could be shared with another child. But at the time it seemed too soon to consider. We did not want to undertake foster parenting with the subconscious motive of replacing our lost child. Besides, our lives, at that point, were too full of grief and turmoil. So we set the idea aside for the time being.

It was not until October of that second year that we decided to take action on the idea. We contacted a private agency that places mentally and physically disabled children and adults in foster homes. After a long process of interviews, documentation, and licensing procedures, we were accepted and certified as a foster family. By this time, we were excited about the prospect of having a new member in our family. But month after month came and went without that prospect being fulfilled. We set our sights on Christmas as a perfect time to welcome a new arrival. But that was not to be.

It was not until February of the new year that we received a phone call on a Friday afternoon. The agency had a five-year-old mentally disabled girl whom they had to place on a short-term, emergency basis, approximately two weeks. She had been through some physical and sexual abuse.

We agreed to take her in. She ended up staying with us for seven and a half months! We have remained a foster family ever since, now with our third long-term placement—an eight-year-old boy who is blind, retarded, and has cerebral palsy.

In caring for children with special needs, we have found both challenge and gratification. It is something we never would have dreamed of doing had we not been given the experience first through David. Though our son never spoke to us, his life did. And we see both our ability and our desire to care for these children as a gift from David, a legacy he left to us. In the role of foster family we have discovered a new and constructive direction for all of us. Though each foster child has been different, each has connected us in some way with David and the sense of purpose he endowed us with. Each one has had his or her own set of hurdles and obstacles that makes them "special". And each one has required of us an unselfish kind of giving that has helped to bring about a healing within us. We know that in caring for them, in providing them with a home and family environment, we are keeping alive the best things that our son gave to us. We are affirming his life as well as ours.

Earlier that same year Barb was offered a part-time job with a grant-funded program called the Family Information Network. David had been enrolled in one of their therapy programs as an infant. Barb's involvement in the program is in helping families of special children. She presents educational workshops that cover the whole spectrum of parenting a special child–from coping emotionally to making decisions for the child. The mission or philosophy behind this program is to build on the strengths already inherent in the family. Barb brings our collective experience to each workshop she presents. This puts her on a common ground with other parents and enables her to relate to the problems, frustrations, achievements, joys and sorrows of special families. Barb has also spoken independently to several groups, both parent and professional, on the experience of losing a disabled child.

Many positive things have blossomed from our loss and our grief. David's short, but eventful, life has shaped our lives profoundly and made us more sensitive, more empathetic, and more responsive to the tragedies in other people's lives. Our long and agonizing journey through the grieving process has changed us. Those profound emotions of sorrow, pain, and depression – and eventual hope and happiness – have become assimilated into the very core of our being, where they have influenced our thoughts, our outlook, our personal growth. It is as though the circumstances, the particularities of our life with David have become rites of passage into a new life, with its own stratems of purpose and design. Though some sorrow remains, it has softened into a sorrow we can live with. There has not been a day gone by that we don't think or daydream about our son. We still ponder our loss, not only in death, but in what he might have been in life. And when we hear the news of the death of a child or some other tragedy striking someone we know, that latent, deep and sharp-edged pain of our own personal loss comes to surface. Someone else's tragedy has often raised those powerful, stirring memories of our own child's death, causing a strong sense of empathy and compassion for the bereaved. It is partly from such events we have learned the lasting effects of our own experience.

David was more than the child we brought into this world and learned to love and accept with all his handicaps. He was a season in our lives, a shattered dream come to fruition. He forced us to grapple deeply with hope and despair, anger, frustration and sorrow, and to search desperately in our hearts and our lives for answers that seemed not to exist. In never speaking to us, in almost never smiling at us, in never extending to us any childish gesture of love or kindness that would inspire a parent to say, "Yes, it is all worth it," he taught us a different kind of love–an unselfish love that can ask little in return. He was the bitter-sweet season, the loss of joy, and the strength to regain it. He drove us apart, then bonded us closer than we'd ever been before. He called forth in us gifts we did not know we had, and a willingness to use them. He brought many wonderful people into our lives whose friendship and support were evident in times both happy and sad. He taught us the importance of "today" everyday. And, finally, he taught us compassion. In these and so many other ways our son's life is validated.

The journey that David took us on was one we would not have chosen for ourselves. In his short life he altered the course of our hopes and dreams, and led us down a path we were certain we could not follow. But somehow we did. And somehow we discovered an inner pride in doing so. In the years since his death we have, each of us, found moments or events when we recognized some good thing within ourselves as a gift from David. In this sense, he affirmed *our* lives. We gave him our hearts. We gave him our love. But he gave us so much more.

Many times, too, my mind has wandered back to that afternoon in the neurologist's office, where he concluded his diagnosis with those ominous words: "I'm afraid this child will not make you very happy." If there is any good and lasting tribute to our son, it is our ability to reflect on those words and say, *How wrong. How wrong he was.*

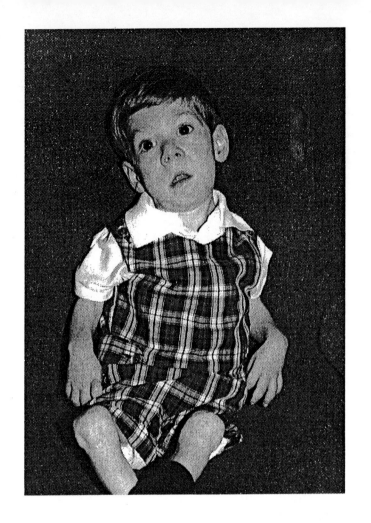

The David
Poems

143

*"So...you must be David.
That's a good name-'David'.
And do you know what it means?
It's a Hebrew word meaning 'beloved
one'."*

A Pediatric Neurologist

You, David

When I see trees
blown and broken,
I think of you, David.

They could not help
themselves against the wind.

Intensive Care

From the hospital window
I can see the first signs of spring:
patches of melting snow,
buds on branches,
young girls walking
their new wardrobes.
Inside, the mood is white
and antiseptic.
Through a maze of tubes and wires
I gaze down at my son,
newborn and baptized,
fallen from heaven.

With the hose in his mouth
he gives this machine a sense of purpose;
it, in turn, gives him breath
to keep the small heart beating
beneath the hand-sewn stitches,
while other tubes empty
their chemicals into him,
mixing a solution called hope.

In this room
in this here and now,
time is severed from reality.
It is measured out
in the beep of monitors,
the drip of intravenous fluids,
the eternal, unanswered question.
And so I wait,
and wait
for an eye to blink,
or a finger to curl,
asking for some hope of heaven,
a god,
a prayer small enough to hold him.

The Silent Ringmaster

I awaken from a dream of fathers and sons
to the sound of my own blood
stirring in another room.
Crossing the moonlight, I open your door,
but you have as quickly fallen
back asleep. Motionless.
Your fastened eyelids hold off the light.
What lies behind them
twists the day into memory?...
perception?..nothing?
Does darkness, for you,
burn brighter than day?

Your room is like a circus tent,
filled with the things
your mother has done to brighten it:
on your dresser
a night-light clown sells balloons
that glow with electric color;
the unicycle
hanging from a ceiling corner
sends another clown wheeling
across some invisible tightrope;
up the wall
a hot air balloon
lifts its furry passengers
beneath a sculptured rainbow.

And on the shelf above your bed
a menagerie of stuffed animals
huddles in stunned silence--
the lion, the elephant,
bulldog and bears,
some with music in their bellies.
They hold their quiet vigil

over you, the keeper,
the silent ringmaster.

What they glimpse with their plastic eyes
blazes back at me
like the echo of a question
whispered over and over
in this same still room:
"What thoughts, what dreams
can flare in the head
where so much brain is useless?"
What wonder for this child
who cannot imagine a circus?

Oh, my son, what I would give
to move behind the blueness of your eyes,
to assemble the fragments of sight and sound,
to make the animals come alive.
I would rise up like a ringmaster
and crack the whip
that sends the lion roaring
through rings of fire,
or the elephant standing on one hind leg,
or bears --many bears --
dancing in an awkward circle.
All sound! All color! All motion
coming together in mid-brain
with whip-snapping clarity!

And the painted clown would turn
his somersaults and handstands,
baggy legs kicking in the air.
The fisted bulldog would strut on two feet.
The balloon would rise higher,
and higher still,
taking on a rainbow of colors,
while another clown scrambles
up the fearsome pole

toward the high wire
thrumming in your head.

And you, my child, would be amazed
by this greatest show on earth,
your gaze becoming sharpened
and meaningful,
enthralled by the shapes appearing,
the air spinning into pure light,
the instant flickering of colors
you did not know existed.
Every nerve vaulting!
Every synapse joining!
Every pulsing message reaching
the failed brain!

Your palsied hands coming suddenly
together in applause,
understanding, for a moment,
the mystery of symmetry, poise and power
here beneath the big top:
where the ringmaster's heart stands
up kingly inside him,
where a child's wonder
is suspended in awesome balance,
like the spoked wheel
flashing on the wire,
like the elephant on one leg,
like the whole circus,
singing and weeping
in our heads.

A Blessing

The house this morning is quiet.
Sitting at the breakfast table,
holding you,
and sipping the last drops
of the morning's coffee,
I feel a special closeness to you.
The way you fit
neatly and comfortably
in the crook of my arm,
your small face,
your slack, open-mouthed expression,
and the wide innocence of your eyes
all speak of a love
you are unable to express—
only to sense
in some remote way
that I will never understand.

But in this beautiful moment of silence,
I accept the incomprehensible
gift you have given me.
I celebrate your being,
my heart opening
like the petals of a new blossom.

In the Light of Day

It is easy in the light of day
to accept those things my son will never do.
Lord knows, I've done it many times.
Today was no different.
At the family picnic he was passed
from one lap to another,
cuddled and stroked.
In a glance, I saw his hair
turn amber in the afternoon sun,
his eyes staring blankly
over the soft sway of his grandmother's shoulder.
The moment lifted me
like a benediction.

Evening has come.
At home now, he lies in darkness,
remembering nothing of the day.
In another room
I sit beside the darkened window
and let the day come back,
knowing what it brings.

There is a certain joy felt only
by fathers at play with their children.
I saw it this afternoon.
My brother chased his toddling son
on the grass beneath a maple.
Now here,
now there,
the falsetto squeal,
the small legs churning below the diapered rump,
he circled,
wide-eyed and giggling,
beyond the tree,
out into greener grass, brighter sunlight,
my brother following.

Together they created a moment
that will come back again
and again through the passages of time.
Tonight they sleep in a lesser darkness,
with the day's play still glowing
in their heads.

Where is that moment for me,
for my son who cannot run,
who sees grass as merely a color,
hears laughter as merely a noise?
What will I give him for memories?
And where will he keep them?
Questions I ask of the darkness.

Tonight I will walk my heart,
with its longing for answers,
out under stars
to pray for children like my own
for fathers who dreamed
of perfect sons, and got less,
and therefore weep in darkness,
longing for morning,
because it is easy,
easy in the light of day.

The music in my heart I bore long after it was heard no more
William Wordsworth
"The Solitary Reaper"

Morning Circle
(for Penny and Kathy)

To give a name to ritual
is to somehow define it.
For two women who teach my son
it is called the "morning circle:"
an arrangement of chairs--
some with legs,
some with straps and wheels.
In the middle of this circle
they lead the seated children in song,
each child accompanying
with a jangling instrument or noisemaker.
Some can barely hold them.
One teacher helps my son
grasp the tambourine
and shake its rings of hammered tin
into rhythm.

Are rhythm and song lost
on children who grope for a voice
to sing, to wail, to moan?
A helpless choir,
out of tune, out of time.
A noisy rhapsody
played out through laughter and smiles.
The broken notes of clashing music
strung together
only by the melody of two voices
that do not stop
for one breathless moment
trying to break through,
to fill their minds with sounds
that connect from the body.
A song their heads can keep.

A song that gathered me, one day,
like a true believer,
into the congregation of that failing circle
to pass beyond myself
into voice.

Fellow believers,
I have seen the morning descend
on a ring of imperfect children.
I have heard the dissonant sounds
risen from shaken hands
and inadequate voices.
I have felt, in my own soul,
the power of their resonant discord
that defies anyone
to call it anything
other than what it truly is:
music.

Artist Unknown
(for David)

The teacher at the county facility
    sends my son's artwork
    home with him.
Today was fingerpainting.
And neatly folded in the blue
    vinyl bag that rides
the bus with him each day

he has brought me a rainbow
    spanning from a cloud
    of glued-on cotton balls.
He is unaware of the gift
    he has given me,
or of the strange mingling
    of pride and pain
    with which I receive it,

knowing it is not really
    his own creation,
but, rather, the design
of a teacher, a therapist--
whoever moved the helpless hand
across a blank sheet of paper.

For this is the unknown artist,
    the child for whom
    there are no choices--
    only colors
emblazoned on a blue paper sky
by the guided, paint-dipped hand
    moving slowly
through the unstudied curves.

In reinventing something
    he has never perceived,

was he surprised at the arc-
like motion of his own hand
across the make-believe sky?
Did he wonder
at the suffusion of colors
that flowed from his fingers?
Did those colors glisten in his eyes?
Shimmer in his head?
The questions themselves are eternal,
unanswered, unanswerable.
They are what fasten
this rainbow to a wall in our home
and keep its bright, banded colors
blazing in my mind.

And yet, this child,
who pressed his hand against the sky
and set it ablaze
with stroke after stroke
of tremendous color,
left his mark amidst
the manipulated lines and swirls:
the whorls and creases
of two small fingers
where they stopped
at the end of a rainbow.

They stand as a kind of self portrait,
a statement by the artist
proclaiming once and for all
that he exists,
that the true purpose of art
is reason
enough for rainbows.

And what better place for a rainbow
than here,
where rain has fallen deeply,

where love, sorrow, and tenderness
hold together
like a cloud that enfolds the heart--

a cloud split suddenly,
almost joyfully,
by a brilliant spectrum
of sky-bending hues;
because the unchosen paints
glowed into colors
that took their shape and meaning
from the hand of a half-brained child,
an unknown artist:
my son,
my gentle son.

Two Hands and a Heart
(Valentine's Day, 1985)

On the refrigerator door
hangs the gift
from a son who has no sense
of his mother's pain:
the white tracings of two small hands
glued to a red paper heart.
She praises the pale hands
in their awkward arrangement,
and the uneven scribble
of the name above them--
"David".

No amount of therapy will shift those hands
to their intended symmetry,
or straighten the name scrawled
across the heart's balanced lobes.
No amount of love will bring
to his mouth the words
a mother yearns to hear.

Knowing this, she accepts it.
Accepting it, she bends
to lift him from the straps of his chair,
to press him close, and to give him
the gift he so thoughtlessly,
so innocently gave to her:
two hands and a heart.

There Are No Words

Fathers and sons can walk
together for a little while,
before love's bonding language
of laughter and play
gives way to other interests.
I walk my own son
out in the back yard,
where we have buried all hope
of sharing a spoken language.
Instead, we share our voices.
He curls toward the sound of mine.
I hearken to his coos and moans.
We pretend to understand.

I carry his helpless body
across the lawn
to a place where we probe the vines
for fruit hidden among the leaves.
A ripened grape squeezed
above his slackened mouth
is something he knows of joy.
And if my son could speak,
he would tell you there are no words
for the juice of the grape
bursting its skin,
trickling to the lip and tongue,
or the feel of the breeze touching
our faces, filling our lungs,
our hair, our silence...
But he has no words.

Whatever the wind says,
it speaks for both of us.

Water
(for Marion)

One photograph,
and I can dream my son back
to something he loved:

A teacher at his side
like the warm wetness of water,
her hands free
and there for him,
she floats him gently
among the blue ripples of the pool.
Trusting those hands
and the water's warm embrace,
the palsied muscles relax.
He is buoyed up,
becoming the slight motion of water,
forgetting what he is,
but knowing where.
And she moves the spindly limbs
in gestures of mercy,
speaking to him softly.
Together they share a balance,
a fellowship born of water and compassion.

Years beyond that picture,
I would cup my hands
beneath a faucet
and watch it weep through my fingers.

Years beyond that picture,
the same woman who held him floating
would come to comfort us,
and I would see it again --
something unstoppable
running through her memory,
filling her,
rising in her eyes:
water, water.

Burial

In the shade of the arborvitae
our priest invokes a simple truth:
unto dust we shall return.
Your mother, your brother, your sister
    and I
join the solemn requiem of words
in the late sun of a summer's end.
Each of us, in turn,
blesses the tiny box --
all that remains of you --
with a sprinkling of water
in a crossing motion.
And so your ashes are laid to rest
among the dust of others.

The prayers ended,
your brother and sister let go
their heart-shaped balloons,
each with a message tethered to its string.
We stand on this ground
where you lie now, deeper than life,
and watch their hopeful rising,
their flash and flicker in the sunlit silence.
They are beautiful in their floating,
shifting on currents of air,
ascending quickly through the earth's
    own breath,
up over treetops, through layer after layer
of clouds – then utterly gone
toward some measureless moment,
some indefinable blue,
like you, my son,
like you.

Only What We Can

All darkness.
In the midnight of our sorrow
we lie on our separate pillows like stones.
There is no solace in this bed
where our loss was conceived years ago.
Your hand searches the mattress for mine.
They join. They bridge the distance
between us, but not in us.

Who are we now, having given
a child to the earth?
So broken we cannot comfort each other.
You hear my sobs.
I know your eyes are filling.
But what words, what gestures can we offer
that have not already been spoken or given?
How do we bear the burden
of a changed world like lovers?
And what comes after this silence,
when our fingers let go
and we stare into darkness?

We are learning the quiet language
of grief -- not words, but sounds
the heart makes in breaking;
not embraces, but the tentative touch
of two hands in the night;
not oneness, but a common aloneness.

This sad, strange language
is all we have to navigate
through the gray gathering of emotions.
So we study it for now, for our own sakes,
for the sake of our dead son:
we learn, we understand,
we give to each other
only what we can.

Kneeling

I have swept the fresh clippings
of grass from his grave,
and traced the bronze letters
of his name with my hand.
Years ago I knelt like this,
an altar boy with a head-
ful of prayers and a child's vision
of heavenly hosts, choirs of angels
kneeling before the fiery throne
of heaven ablaze with glory.
But somewhere I stood up
and became a mortal man,
a husband, a father
called to the things of this world
by love and necessity,
then brought to his knees again
by what God has given
and taken away.

What a strange theology
to balance the death of a child
with a loving and merciful God.
A contradiction of the heart.
A logic that bends the mind,
bends the body at the knees
in an attitude of devotion
that defies all reason.

Something inside me rises
like a prayer I cannot enter,
too burdened with my own thoughts
and the memory of a small face.
And yet I stay here,
with my knees to the earth
and everything inside of me kneeling,
searching for words to call
down some god, some angel,
some spirit bathed in heavenly light
to lift me beyond what is here,
to comfort me, to touch me,
to whisper to me softly,
I know. I know.

Beauty and Sadness

A child is lost,
and all the world's beauty
becomes soluble.
Sights and sounds
that once held your breath
now wash over you
like a wave of sorrow.
You can stand in a winter snowfield
or walk a wooded path in springtime,
you can hear music
or the sounds of children at play,
but are no longer lifted.
Blinded and voiceless,
you wonder how this world,
with its beauty so awesome and subtle,
can compass such tragedy.

This is the equation few have known:
that beauty and sadness are two
sides of the same coin.
It is the purity of sorrow,
the poverty of spirit
for those who dig deep
into the heart's empty pocket,
possessing nothing but that coin
rolled and pressed between the fingers
over and over again.

9 - 19 - 87

Out in the yard
everything looks unchanged.
The willow stands tall and graceful
in the morning sun.
Bees are thrumming around
the ripe, neglected fruit
beneath the pear tree.
Two rabbits graze between
burned-out patches of summer grass.
And the fiery heads of your mother's flowers
are nodding toward another season.

It is September, one month after
your death, and I am standing
under the maple's spreading arms
saying your name.
Looking around, I bless every leaf,
every blade of grass,
every color that may
have caught your eye
or filled you with wonder.
David, I am walking.

I am walking to places in the yard
where I carried you.
And every step brings a snapshot memory:
you in summer's brightest colors;
you at the swingset,
swinging on your sister's lap;
you on the tractor,
riding the rugged lawn
in your mother's arms;
and our after-dinner strolls,
our one-sided conversations.

Sometimes, wide-eyed and open-mouthed,
you arched your small neck
to wonder at clouds...
or blueness...or something.

David, I am walking
through the yard that no longer sings
since darkness fell upon you.
It is another country now,
and I a melancholy traveler
as lost today as the days to come.
The damp morning is silent.
The sun's risen light
falls across the lawn
and burns everything into being,
the way I wish my voice could do,
speaking your name.

But the sun is a power beyond me,
a reminder of the things I cannot do,
like send the greenness springing
into the grass again,
or hang the rotting fruit
perfect on its branches.
I can only arch my neck
to wonder at the sky
and search with the eyes of a hopeless poet
for that one metaphor
that would transcend your life and death
and hold you gently
floating in time.

David, I am walking.

The Small Things

All night a tree branch scratches
against the window screen
like a thought that will not leave.
Morning finds me standing
beside the bed wondering
why I have risen. What will I do?

The sounds of the world going on
are distant. I move through silences
in the rooms of your lost life.
Everywhere the reminders of you:

In the kitchen cupboard jars
of baby food are stacked
alongside the coffee.
Beside them, your spoon, your warming dish.
In the family room your wide blue eyes
gaze out from framed photographs.
A still life of innocence.
And in your bedroom, the empty crib,
the rows of folded white diapers
waiting to wrap you,
the look of bewilderment
on the faces of stuffed animals.

David, I mourn the small things –
these things that refuse to die
as quickly as you.
I save them.
I come into these rooms to imagine
you, to breathe in solitary spaces
that once held your presence.
And I pray to the small things
to give back whatever
can be salvaged from memory.
Forever. Forever.
How fiercely I cling
to what I cannot hold.

The Grieving

"Life must go on,"
they tell us,
"Time will heal."
But time is the distance
that separates,
the silence swelling within us,
the gulf we stare across each day,
the shadow growing long and longer.

And isn't there something precious
in this mourning
that makes us want to stop
time before our grief dissolves,
and we have nothing,
nothing left?

Where I Stand

Two months later
I am looking for your window,
where I stand
on the hospital sidewalk.
I see it now,
glinting in the afternoon light
like something outside of time.
Behind its glass
hovers the process of things
I cannot grasp or hold.

David, I want to go back
up to that room.
I want to empty myself
and float upward
through sunlight and glass
into that room where your lungs gave out,
the room that still holds my memory.

I want to stand in the numbing silence
and remember.
I want to breathe that close air
and hold it deep,
until my own two lungs
swell like balloons
holding deep
where I stand staring
at these empty arms
that cradled your death.
Let heart and memory play together
like two small children,
and I see with my innermost eye
the doctor shaking his head,
the sympathetic nurse explaining
how you will go peacefully.
Holding deep, deeper.

I can hear inside me
the terrible silence of machines.
Then a moment comes on--
piercing, breathless, intensified--
when everything about you is fading
and failing, your life
lifting gently, letting go.
Holding! Holding!
Breath! Heartbeat! Nothing
but a quiet beyond belief.

My son, I would rise
from the stillness of your death
to walk to that window
and let go this grief-keeping,
lung-bursting breath,
to look down through the steamed glass
and see my own self looking up:
renewed, made whole once again
in your beautiful shining
on this sidewalk
where I stand
breathing.

"And with the morn, those angel faces smile
Which I have loved long since, and lost awhile "
John Henry, Cardinal Newman

Angels in the Snow

Too wise for the comings and goings of angels,
I am turned by their laughter,
to see them lying on their backs
heaving and furling the snow
with their make-believe wings.
Against the immeasurable whiteness
my son and daughter look so small,
so luminous
they could pass for heavenly creatures.

I lie down between them
and mimic that celestial motion
that transfigures each of us into angels.
They touch me with the tips of their wings
as though bearing me up
through a sorrow that holds time.
Having counted too much on miracles
and perfection of prayers that hover
in my silence, I find all things
in their form are fragile and fleeting.
We flail our arms
as if the figures they shape
have some purpose or permanence.
But these soft castings we make in snow
will glaze and melt
and leave no hint of us.

As I beat my blessed wings,
I think of an angel who passed from this earth,
whose frail wings
lifted him before his time
and left a soft impression
that will not melt,
who never spoke a word or uttered a prayer,
and whom I called, however briefly,
son.

In the Living Room

She knows the music like a dream:
those Strauss waltzes that played on the stereo
and carried him through long afternoons
propped on the living room couch,
a powerless prince on a pillowed throne.

At moments between pain and peace
that music he loved comes into the air --
or so she imagines...
or perhaps the music imagines itself...
imagines her in the living room
filling her emptiness with sound.

Hearing it, she can dream
the shape of his being there
on the couch, unreachable now.
The Emperor Waltz, The Blue Danube,
The Voices of Spring play on
through the afternoon's calm procession.
Like him, she does not study them.
She knows only that they fill
a longing, a dark place in the brain,
the way they bloomed inside of his.

Sweet music, indeed, for a child
who could not pass the hours at play,
for a mother who listens in measured time
and loses herself
in a room that holds nothing,
nothing but a song.

The Hues of Winter

The father-dreamer walks a path along the river
on a day that could be any other day.
It is February. The river is ice.
He tries to remember a season with its leaves
so thick and shiny. That day he strapped
his small son to his back the river moved
like time slowly beside them.
And the path was a cool corridor,
arched and green, where the sun peeked through
the crooks of branches and dappled down
through the hollow spaces of leaves.
"Ah, what color!" he told his speechless boy.

He can't believe his son's been dead for months,
or how memories warm and cool the winter.
If he walks far enough, if he dreams hard enough,
will that season of human time come back
to inhabit him for a little while?
Can his shoulders, his back, his feet imagine
the weight of another now gone?
He stops to stare at the river, the frozen landscape,
as if looking in a mirror. The hues of winter
are the hues of memory: black and white,
a soft gray along the snowy banks.
"Ah, what color," he says to no one.

Mourning Ritual

In a room where sunlight steals
in from the edge of a windowshade,
a father waits
for his child's waking sound.
But the room is silent.
He leaves the chair
to stand beside the crib.
But the crib is empty.
He leans over the side to lift
the emptiness and hold it,
nuzzle it neck to neck,
and to carry it down the hallway
asking the same question
he always asked,
but now in a whisper
that sounds like a prayer:
"How's my boy this morning?"

Sleeping on the Floor in My Son's Bedroom

Looking up through the moonlit darkness,
I see the striped, parallel shadows
of your crib against the wall,
and the bold silhouette
of the rocking horse I built
with these hands.
You never rode it.
Yet, I think of the times
in your short life you rocked
so close to the edge;
nothing but doctors, drugs,
our own vulnerable prayers
brought you back each time.

David, you are two years gone
and have no need
of medicine or prayers.
So what can a father do,
missing his son?
What can a father do,
whose hand still remembers
the day your heart
relaxed beneath it?
In the stillness of this empty room
there are no answers.

So I lie down in darkness,
hoping for what only
the night can give me:
a moment still and sacred enough
to gather grief and sorrow,
courage and strength enough
to mount the dark
horse of memory,
and rock gently on the edge
between past and present,
sleeping and waking,
my hand tingling
beneath my head.

Making Ready the Room

Starting out, we are mostly silent,
speaking only of details
and what must be done.
We are making ready the room,
now vacant,
for a child from the county
who needs a family.

I dismantle the crib.
My wife empties the closet,
the drawers, the changing table,
folding each article with a kind of reverence,
placing it in a clean box.
"Remember this sweater?...these shoes?"
she asks, holding out
item after item in front of her,
a fashion show of memories.
I nod. I say "My God,
he was a handsome boy."
Then back to work.

Strange how death renders things useless --
furniture, clothing, a rocking horse --
yet how each is raised
to the dignity of a sacred object
because it somehow connects
to the child now gone.

It is the right thing we are doing,
this packing and storing of memories,
though we feel like vandals
desecrating some holy place.
But our grief has brought us this far:
no longer to weep or question why,
but merely to bend,
to pick up boxes,
to raise them shoulder-high.

Beyond

In the counterpointing of hope and despair
I have tried to balance your life and death.
But the scale is tipped by times remembered.
I love your life more now than ever.

Your brief moment has turned my days
to darkness, then back to light. It flickers
like candle-glow in every corner of my mind.
It shines and shapes my days.

But nothing brings you back, my son.
Everything calls me toward your life --
that gift you have given, that poem that fills me
and becomes the way I move and bend.

If this is what must be, then let your death
impart some purpose. Let it gather me,
connect me, and empower me to take
my steps beyond the sorrow of today.

As I pass through this place I have not been,
Let me know the things you touched, that touched
you.
Let me call them longings or blessings.
I will walk this way the rest of my life.

I love your life more now than ever.
It shines and shapes my days,
and becomes the way I move and bend
my steps beyond the sorrow of today.
I will walk this way the rest of my life.

Listening to the Tree
(Spring, 1989)

Your mother turned a circle in the earth
and planted flowers around this tree
the neighbors brought in your name.
Last week the sleeping buds opened
like a secret held too long,
and draped it in foliage of dark red.
The slender trunk of the flowering plum
has thickened, the branches grown out.
Under the sun it stands silent and motionless,
dreaming of soft rains, another summer.

It does not forget the sad season
of its planting, but contains it,
wraps it in a rind of rippled bark,
pressing into pith and heartwood,
those rings of time.
It goes on growing as though it had
no choice. Leaves gathering, multiplying
in the branches. Roots pulling down,
fastening, nourishing cell by cell
the distance from trunk to leaftip,
dreaming in the dark earth
a dream of size and strength.

David, there are no tears.
The tree has spoken,
saying we are all earth. I have listened
to its strong and subtle gestures,
studied the grace of branch and leaf.
And this morning I lift my face.
I lean into deep crimson—
those leaves clustered like jewels—
and I whisper to the tree,
saying, "Yes, I see what you mean."

Looking Down

There comes a time when the wire
you are walking grows slack.
A swaying motion sets in.
You look down
between outstretched arms,
your whole body trembling
with the question, "What if...?"
And your only balance coming
from the risks you weigh in each hand.
Turn around?   Go forward?
One as dangerous as the other.
Then suddenly, you shrug
your shoulders, you laugh,
you place one foot in front
of the other, then again...
again...

The author, Bob Greenwald, is a member of the National Fathers' Network. The Foreword to this book was written by the Program Director of the National Fathers' Network.

The National Fathers' Network, with over 6,000 members throughout the world, advocates for fathers and families of children with chronic illnesses and developmental disabilities. Funded through a grant from the Maternal and Child Health Bureau, the NFN is the only national program fully committed to providing effective, invaluable supports and resources for fathers, and to promoting fathers as important, caring people involved in the lives of their special children. Outreach services of the Network include:

♦ sharing ideas, concerns and resources
♦ developing father support and mentoring programs
♦ developing curriculum, monographs and videos for fathers and fathers' groups
♦ assisting professionals in developing inclusive "father-friendly" services in health care delivery systems
♦ tri-yearly publication of DADS (Dads Advocating for Dads), a newsletter written and produced by fathers
♦ a monthly column in *Exceptional Parent* magazine, "Fathers' Voices," read by over 100,000 people

For more information on the National Father's Network, an organization of fathers helping fathers, write to:

National Fathers' Network
Kindering Center
16120 NE Eighth Avenue
Bellevue, WA 98008-3937

or visit the web site at:

http://www.fathersnetwork.org

For information about submitting manuscripts for the People with Disabilities Press, please write: Stanley D. Klein, Ph.D. People with Disabilities Press P. O. Box 470715 Brookline, MA 02445